BRAIN RESEARCH IN EDUCATION AND THE SOCIAL SCIENCES

Brain Research in Education and the Social Sciences: Implications for Practice, Parenting, and Future Society provides practitioners, parents, and policy makers with research-based information and illustrative case studies about brain development across the lifespan. Neurotechnological advances that are contributing to a broader understanding of brain development and brain illnesses are discussed in a context specifically relevant to those working in education and the social sciences. The book enables readers to understand the societal implications of this expanding knowledge base and offers suggestions for future policies and practices that would make high-quality learning environments available to all students and individuals receiving care.

Doris Bergen is Distinguished Professor of Educational Psychology, Emerita, at Miami University of Ohio, USA.

Joseph Schroer is an educational psychologist and Clinical Professor of Educational Psychology at Miami University of Ohio, USA.

Michael Woodin is a pediatric neuropsychologist and Clinical Professor of School Psychology at Miami University of Ohio, USA.

BRAIN RESEARCH IN EDUCATION AND THE SOCIAL SCIENCES

Implications for Practice, Parenting, and Future Society

Doris Bergen, Joseph Schroer, and Michael Woodin

Routledge
Taylor & Francis Group
NEW YORK AND LONDON

First published 2018
by Routledge
605 Third Avenue, New York, NY 10017

and by Routledge
4 Park Square, Milton Park, Abingdon, Oxon OX14 4RN

Routledge is an imprint of the Taylor & Francis Group, an informa business

Library of Congress Cataloging-in-Publication Data
A catalog record for this book has been requested

ISBN: 978-1-138-20634-2 (hbk)
ISBN: 978-1-138-20635-9 (pbk)
ISBN: 978-1-315-46521-0 (ebk)

Typeset in Bembo
by Apex CoVantage, LLC

To the readers who will use this knowledge to further the optimum development of infants, preschoolers, elementary age children, middle schoolers, adolescents, and adults and prepare them for both the contemporary and the future global society.

CONTENTS

FIGURES

TABLES

INTRODUCTION

Although *Brain Research and Childhood Education: Implications for Educators, Parents, and Society* covered current information about brain research related to child and adolescent brain development, size limitations prevented coverage of adult brain development and information about newer technologies that have expanded knowledge about both typical and atypical brain development. This expanded book version includes the information in *Brain Research and Childhood Education: Implications for Educators, Parents, and Society* as well as these additional issues.

Recently there has been exponential growth in information about structures and functions of the brain and factors influencing brain development at various age levels. Thus, information on the brain's important role in fostering development and learning has expanded. Accurate knowledge about brain structures, functions, and developmental trajectories is useful for professionals working with children, adolescents, and adults, as well as for parents and the general society. It is important to have accurate publications on developmental implications of brain research, rather than publications that assert certain "brain-based" curricula or other materials will "solve" brain development issues (see Bailey et al., 2001; Bruer, 1999; Mareschal, Butterworth, & Tolmie, 2013).

The purpose of this book is to provide research-based information about brain development that informs practitioners, parents, and policy makers because it is no longer possible to consider knowledge of neurobiological processes as lying outside of their areas of expertise. Scientists are not the only ones who need to know how the neuronal network and its communication processes function, and how the brain's modular structures and primary functions are integrated in complex interactions. Although there is more to be learned before direct relationships between brain development and various educational, medical, or societal practices can be clearly demonstrated, both professionals and parents must understand that growth and elaboration of the neuronal network during childhood and adolescence is influential for knowledge construction, and that complex interactions of brain components influence the nature of learning and health throughout life.

Because the brain's plasticity creates multiple opportunities for diverse experiences (or lack of experiences) to influence its development, every educational as well as every other life experience is "brain-based." Each has the potential to influence or be influenced by brain development. Professionals aware of similarities and differences among individual brains should be sensitive to the needs of those whose brains have experienced biological risk, environmental trauma, or human care variability. Families and the larger society need information about neurotechnological methods that explain how brains function and how important healthy environments and positive life experiences are for optimum brain development. This knowledge should help them support practices that make high-quality environments available to all children, adolescents, and adults.

In the first book written on this subject (Bergen & Coscia, 2001), the first author stated three reasons for the need to connect brain research knowledge to practice, and these reasons are still relevant. They are:

1. To inform readers who received their professional training prior to the explosion of brain-related knowledge about the progress in this field.
2. To help readers link their existing development and learning knowledge base to brain research information.
3. To encourage readers to reflect upon present practices, determine if those practices enhance brain development, and incorporate methods informed by knowledge of brain development.

This edition adds two other objectives:

4. To inform readers about neurotechnological advances that are adding to knowledge of brain development, brain illnesses, and suggested treatments.
5. To enable readers to understand societal implications of this expanding knowledge base and offer suggestions for future policies and practices.

Description of the Chapters

Chapter 1 gives an overview of the history of brain research and describes hypotheses that earlier researchers have had about brain structures and functions. It discusses the ways the brain has been studied, advances that have occurred over many years, and more recent methods for studying the brain, as well as the advantages and disadvantages of these methods.

Chapter 2 discusses functions and structures of the brain and gives scientific names of these functions and structures. The information provides the basis for understanding brain development at each age level, and its implications for practice, parenting, and societal decision-making.

Chapters 3–9 focus on different age levels and explain brain development at each age level followed by suggestions for practice related to that stage of brain developmental growth. Possible threats or negative factors that may have an impact on development at each age period also are discussed. Case examples describing issues of brain development at each age level are included and highlight various brain development issues, with discussion of those issues included in the chapter. Implications for families, professional practice, and societal responses also are provided. The chapters conclude with a study guide and questions for discussion.

Chapters 10–12 describe research methods now used to study typical brain development as well as to investigate inherited problems, diseases, and other factors that may result in atypical development. Topics include neuroimaging and neurodiagnostic techniques, electroencephalogram (EEG) and event-related potentials (ERP) methodology, and methods used in clinical and educational practice to understand and potentially influence brain development and functioning. They also include case examples and questions for discussion.

Chapter 13 discusses social policy and educational practice issues that have been related to brain development and often recommended for practice. These are evaluated in relation to evidence as to whether the practices can be supported by knowledge gained from current brain research.

Chapter 14 reviews issues that may affect human development, education, and social policy in the future and gives suggestions for informed responses to these issues.

Bibliography

Bailey, D. B., Bruer, J. T., Symons, F. J., & Lichtman, J. W. (Eds.). (2001). *Critical thinking about critical periods*. Baltimore, MD: Paul H. Brookes.

Bergen, D., & Coscia, J. M. (2001). *Brain research and childhood education: Implications for educators*. Olney, MD: Association for Childhood Education International. [Translated and published in China, 2006]

Bruer, J. T. (1999, May). In search of . . . brain-based education. *Phi Delta Kappan*, 649–657.

Mareschal, D., Butterworth, B., & Tolmie, A. (Eds.). (2013). *Educational neuroscience*. New York: John Wiley & Sons.

1

UNDERSTANDING THE BRAIN

> Men ought to know that from the brain, and from the brain only, arise our pleasures, joys, laughter and jests, as well as our sorrows, pains, griefs and tears. Through it, in particular, we think, see, hear, and distinguish the ugly from the beautiful, the bad from the good, the pleasant from the unpleasant . . . it . . . makes us mad or delirious, inspires us with dread or fear, whether by night or by day, brings sleeplessness, inopportune mistakes, aimless anxieties, absent-mindedness, and acts that are contrary to habit.
>
> —Hippocrates
>
> *The Sacred Disease*, in *Hippocrates*, Trans. W. H. S. Jones (1923), Vol. 2, 175

A Brief History of the Study of the Brain

Recent emphasis on brain research suggests that study of the brain is a new phenomenon; however, structures and functions of the brain have been studied by physicians, philosophers, and researchers since earliest times. Archeologists have found what appears to be the deliberate drilling of holes in human skulls, perhaps to relieve pressure from brain injury. As early as 1700 BC, Egyptian doctors used surgery to treat brain injuries and observed connections between the central nervous system, sensation, and locomotion. In the mummification process, however, Egyptians preserved the heart and liver but not brain matter (Finger, 1994, 2001). Most information about the human brain was based upon study of dead animals and humans, so many assumptions about the human brain were erroneous. (e.g., human and sheep brains had similar cavities).

In 450 BC, Alcmaeon of Croton described the optic nerve as being a path of light to the brain (Gross, 1998). Early interest in the brain was evident in China, India, and Syria from 400 BC to 100 AD (Finger, 1994, 2001; Gross, 1998). The Chinese stated there was a connection between the eyes and the brain (i.e., the evil eye), and Nemesius of Syria proposed that basic sensory and motor functions were in the ventricles (cavities). This (incorrect) view was accepted throughout the middle ages. Greek and Roman philosophers and physicians also debated functions of the brain. Hippocrates drilled holes in the skulls of patients because he thought it would balance the humours of the brain and Galen identified the autonomic and sympathetic nervous systems, stating that wounds of the brain affect the mind. However, he concluded that the outer portion of the brain (the cortex) was just a covering with no functional importance ("cortex" means "rind" or "bark"). Although Plato saw the brain as the site of sensation and thought, Aristotle thought the heart was the major center of rationality and that the brain only cooled "humours" of the blood. This "cardiocentric" view prevailed throughout the middle ages. Aristotle stated that "spirit" circulated freely in the brain, via *sensus communis*, which came to be known as "common sense."

Beginnings of Scientific Study

Prior to the thirteenth century, most physicians were associated with the Church, so doctors applied a mix of religious dogma and medicinal practices to brain injuries and diseases (Finger, 2001). In the mid-fourteenth century, most serious injuries (e.g., during wars) were not treated, as it was thought humours would be released into the brain, which, being untreatable, would kill the person. By the mid-1500s, medicine began to be based on anatomy and physiology, and physicians operated on severe head injuries with surgical tools and pharmacological means (Finger, 2001). Vesalius concluded that Galen's earlier description of brain anatomy was erroneous and suggested revisions. Leonardo da Vinci's illustrations of animal brains and his wax casts of brain ventricles offered precise anatomical information about brain structures and, although his information corrected earlier illustrations of the brain, it still did not challenge the incorrect idea that the ventricles were sources of sensory and motor functions.

The Renaissance opened a new world of brain study (Finger, 1994; Gross, 1998). Systematic study of relationships between brain and learning processes began in the seventeenth and eighteenth centuries. Using the microscope (an early technological advance), Malpighi studied the anatomy of the cortex, Willis suggested that the gyri (bulging folds of the cerebral cortex) controlled memory and will, and Descartes identified the pineal gland while still asserting that the brain and the mind were two different entities (Gross, 1998). By the 1700s, various areas of the brain had been identified as responsible for specific functions. For example, Legallois isolated the medulla as the respiratory center of the brain (Cheung, 2013), Swedenborg identified separate motor and sensory cortical areas (Fingers, 1994), Flourens reported that the cerebellum coordinated movement (Yildirim & Sarikcioglu, 2007), Broca showed that motor control of language was in the frontal cortex (Pierre-Paul Broca, 2000), and Wernicke identified the temporal lobe as the site for interpretation of spoken language (Finger, 1994).

Unfortunately, Gall's promotion of phrenology, an incorrect view asserting that skull shape and features were related to personality characteristics, gained prominence until it was attacked by Flourens, who stated that the brain acts as a whole to form intelligence. Although still discussed in some introductory psychology courses, phrenology was discounted by the late 1800s.

Prior to the 1900s, with the assistance of electrophysical recordings (another technological advance), Cajal established the "Neuron Doctrine," stating that neurons were independent units composed of cell bodies, axons, and dendrites; Schwann identified the myelin sheaths (fat-like deposits) on neurons; and Sherrington found the "spaces" between axon and dendrites (the synapses) and studied how messages were transmitted across the synapses (Finger, 1994, 2001; Gross, 1998; Yuste, 2015). By the early 1900s, the theory that brain functions were specific to certain areas was challenged by the equipotentiality theory, which suggested that all areas of the brain contribute equally to behaviors (Lashley, 1950). Lashley later modified his theory to suggest that subareas of each region have some specific functions. Luria (1973) developed a competing idea of the brain as being composed of "functional systems," which suggested that multiple areas of the brain function together to produce behaviors. Franz first investigated the brain's relationship to learning by studying the brain's ability to learn or relearn after it had been damaged (Finger, 1994, 2001). His findings suggested that new pathways could be developed after brain injury, supporting more integrated theories of brain functioning.

During the late twentieth century, major technological advances enabled brain researchers to engage in more precise study of the brain. The development of metabolic, electrophysiologic, magnetic, and neuropsychological methods for studying living brains has enabled researchers to learn much more about relationships between brain structures and functions (Zillmer, Spiers, & Culbertson, 2008). Information in this book is primarily derived from research using these newer procedures. They include metabolic procedures such as positron emission tomography (PET), single photon emission tomography (SPECT), and functional magnetic resonance imaging (fMRI); electrophysiological procedures such as EEG and ERP; and magnetic procedures such as magnetic source imaging (MSI), magnetic encephalography (MEG), and diffusion tensor imaging (DTI). Because the procedures are still being refined and extended, many of the implications of these findings for education and development are hypotheses only. The advantages and disadvantages of each procedure are shown in Table 1.1.

Metabolic Procedures

These procedures permit researchers to learn more about *where* thinking is occurring in the brain. They include positron emission tomography (PET), single-photon emission tomography (SPECT), and functional magnetic resonance imaging (fMRI). PET and SPECT procedures follow the flow and usage of radioactive

TABLE 1.1 Advantages and Disadvantages of Current Brain Research Techniques

Technique	*Advantages*	*Disadvantages*
PET/SPECT Positron emissions tomography/single-photon emission tomography	—Non-invasive —Able to localize brain activity —Able to use on young children	—Ethical questions of use of radioactive materials on the young —Range of isolation of activity is centimeter range (not precise) —Brief time span before decay of signal —Expensive
fMRI Functional magnetic resonance imaging	—Noninvasive —No exposure to radiation —Precise; isolates areas in range of millimeters —Fast	—Participants must be very still —High level of noise may be painful —Cramped environment —Expensive
EEG Electroencephalogram	—Noninvasive —Sensitive to state changes —Relatively inexpensive	—Gives general information; not really suited to study of cognitive processes —Poor spatial and temporal resolution
ERP Event-related potentials	—Can examine cognitive activity —Each signal marked by specific event/stimulus, so more accurate temporal information —More electrodes, so more accurate spatial information —Many measures in brief time	—Errors occur if extraneous movement (muscles, eyes), resulting in loss of trial or cases
MSI/MEG Magnetic source imaging/ encephalography	—Fast enough to track neural signals —Tracks neural pathways directly —Yields good spatial (in millimeters) and temporal (in milliseconds) data	—Only reads signals near brain surface —Extremely sensitive to outside magnetic fields (moving metal objects) —Expensive
DTI Diffusion tensor imaging	—Noninvasive —More sensitive to white matter injury of the brain than other imaging techniques —Highly sensitive to tears in white matter or diffuse axonal injury (DAI) —Can be used along with neuropsychological testing to show evidence of cognitive decline —Can help predict recovery times for concussion patients	—Similar to other MRI tests —Expensive —Highly sensitive to distortion based on movement by the patient —Images can be blurry due to its low spatial resolution

Technique	*Advantages*	*Disadvantages*
Neuropsychological assessment	—Noninvasive —Tasks can be used in animal research to make inferences about human behavior —Can be used with children and across lifespan	—Most tools measure more than one behavior, so difficult to isolate behaviors —Difficult to determine precise location of brain lesion or dysfunction

compounds (e.g., oxygen or glucose for PET and technetium-99 or xenon-133 for SPECT) through the brain while the person is performing mental tasks. As the radioactive substance decays, a positron (positively charged electron-like particle) is emitted and tracked. High emissions from an area means high levels of oxygen or glucose are required in that area during cognitive activity; therefore, the areas of greatest activity during particular tasks (e.g., naming pictures, reading, memorizing) can be observed.

Chugani and colleagues used PET scans with infants in the early and mid-1990s, making important foundational inferences about the rapid synaptic development during infancy and childhood (e.g., Chugani, Phelps, & Mazziota, 1993). More recently, Chugani and colleagues have used PET combined with MRI data to confirm hypotheses about the finding that the rate of glucose uptake by the brain does not peak at birth, when the size of the brain relative to the body is largest, but in childhood, when synaptic densities and related metabolic processes are maximal (Kuzawa et al., 2014). This finding suggests that "humans evolved a protracted period of slow pre-adult growth to compensate for the unusually high metabolic costs of brain development underlying the extraordinary human capacity for cultural learning" (Kuzawa et al., 2014). Further discussion of these procedures is in Chapter 10.

Electrophysiologic Procedures

These procedures are used to explore the question of *when* thinking is occurring. They include electroencephalogram (EEG) and event-related potentials (ERP). In the EEG procedure, electrodes fastened to the scalp monitor and record the electrical activity of the brain: a byproduct of neuronal communication. This procedure has informed diagnosis and treatment of children with seizure disorders like epilepsy (Wyllie et al., 1998). Recently, EEG techniques have been used to predict the onset of seizures and have led to newer technologies, allowing families to monitor the onset of seizures at home (van Andel et al., 2016). Seizures are also studied by ERP research using scalp-fastened electrode procedures and flashing stimuli in front of subjects, and monitoring the resultant electrical activity in the brain. Benasich and Spitz (1998) used ERP to study children's language development and found that later language disorders could be predicted based on ERP findings in infancy. ERP-based methods and research are further described in Chapter 11.

Magnetic Procedures

To explore *where* and *when* thinking is occurring, magnetic source imaging (MSI) and magnetic encephalography (MEG) can be used. The small magnetic field generated by each electrical neural signal can be monitored by superconducting quantum interference devices (SQUIDs), which track the neural signal along its pathway through the brain. Computer analysis of the signals creates a visual map of this pathway. Magnetoencephalography (MEG) takes advantage of the fact that neuromagnetic signals penetrate the skull and scalp without distortion. The magnetic source image (MSI) is created when the MEG data are superimposed on a magnetic resonance image (MRI). These techniques are used in the treatment of multiple conditions, including epilepsy (Wheless et al., 2004), non-lesional epilepsy (Bagić, 2016), sclerosis (Wu et al., 2006), and neurosurgeries (to detect neural circuitry) (Pang & Snead, 2016). Chapter 10 and 12 further discuss these techniques and findings.

Neuropsychological Assessment Procedures

These procedures assume that brain function and behavior are causally related and that neuropsychological measurements can identify behavioral deficits related to brain functioning. Neuropsychological measures refer to tasks (e.g., paper and pencil, oral, performance, computer generated) that examiners administer to patients in a one-on-one setting. These measures test hypotheses about specific brain functions and examine intellectual, memory, attention, language, sensory, motor, visuospatial, and executive functioning. They also focus on academic, social, and behavioral domains. Research in neuropsychological assessment stems from experimental studies of cognitive functions in humans and animals (Lezak, 2004). Recent studies range from the treatment of young children with neurodevelopmental disorders (Racanello et al., 2016) to older adults with Parkinson's disease (Pal et al., 2016). These methods are further discussed in Chapter 12.

Speculative Cognitive Models and Theories of Brain Functioning

Brash, Maranta, Murphy, and Walker (1990) note that the brain is "perhaps alone in all of nature, the only organ that is aware of itself, aware of the universe that surrounds it, aware of life and death" (p. 14). From the research base amassed over many decades, theorists have hypothesized views of the overall function and structure of the brain and of its role in consciousness. Some current brain research investigates rectifying lapses in consciousness after traumatic brain injury (TBI). For example, Monti and colleagues (2016) used low-intensity focused ultrasound pulsation (LIFUP) on the thalamus of a youth who suffered a TBI from a car accident. They report the patient exited the state of coma and began almost normal motor and language function within 19 days from onset of treatment. It is not clear whether the treatment was the cause of the improvement, however.

To understand different functions of the brain more clearly, better understanding of the structures of the brain is needed. Brain mapping involves neuroscience techniques that plot biological quantities or properties of the brain onto spatial representations of the brain, resulting in "maps." Mapping the normal brain's structure and function is helpful in many areas, including treatment and control of seizures in children with brain tumors (Berger et al., 1989; Liang & Wang, 2017). Recently, Harvey and Dumoulin (2016) used fMRI techniques to create topographical maps of the adult brain during a numeracy task. They theorized that networks of neurons combine to create representations of numerosity in the same way that neuron networks dedicated to the visual field create complex responses to visual stimuli. Development and dissemination of topographical maps is important for two reasons. First, because most neural processing is context dependent, brain maps help clinicians and researchers to focus on specific areas of the brain for treatment. Second, brain mapping provides researchers with the ability to compare and contrast results with other context maps, leading to more informed hypotheses that focus research in specific areas of the brain.

In the twenty-first century, methods for studying the brain have become more sophisticated, and continuing advances have led to greater knowledge of how brains are able to (as Hippocrates observed) "think, see, hear, and distinguish the ugly from the beautiful, the bad from the good, the pleasant from the unpleasant." However, although most brain *structures* have been defined in detail, there are many aspects of brain *functions* that still are not clearly understood and remain important areas of research. Many current studies focus on understanding precise ways that these functions occur within various interacting brain structures. Other researchers investigate how brain functions and structures are related to mental health conditions similar to those of concern to Hippocrates. Current study on the course of brain development (prenatal through adulthood) and the interacting environmental conditions that may foster or hinder optimum development is an especially important aspect for educators, social service professionals, physicians, and parents, and much has been learned in recent years.

Study Guide/Questions for Discussion

- Read an account of a brain study of one of the early brain researchers and describe how that research informed or dis-informed later research.
- Analyze a current brain study using a newer method of research and suggest implications of the findings for education or other professional fields.

Bibliography

Bagić, A. (2016). Look back to leap forward: The emerging new role of magnetoencephalography (MEG) in nonlesional epilepsy. *Clinical Neurophysiology, 127*(1), 60–66.

Benasich, A. A., & Spitz, R. V. (1998). Insights from infants: Temporal processing abilities and genetics contribute to language development. In G. Willems & K. Whitmore (Eds.), *A neurodevelopmental approach to specific learning disorders* (pp. 191–210). London: MacKeith Press.

Berger, M. S., Kincaid, J., Ojemann, G. A., & Lettich, E. (1989). Brain mapping techniques to maximize resection, safety, and seizure control in children with brain tumors. *Neurosurgery, 25*(5), 786–792.

Brash, Maranta, Murphy, and Walker (eds.) (1990). *How Things Work: The Brain.* Alexandria, VA: Time-Life Books.

Cheung, T. (2013). Limits of life and death: Legallois's decapitation experiments. *Journal of the History of Biology, 46*(2), 283–313.

Chugani, H. T., Phelps, M. E., & Massiotta, J. C. (1993). Positron emission tomography study of human brain functional development. In M. H. Johnson (Ed.), *Brain development and cognition: A reader* (pp. 125–143). Oxford: Blackwell.

Finger, S. (1994). History of neuropsychology. In D. Zaidel (Ed.), *Neuropsychology.* San Diego, CA: Academic Press.

Finger, S. (2001). *Origins of neuroscience: a history of explorations into brain function.* New York: Oxford University Press.

Gross, C. G. (1998). *Brain, vision, memory: Tales in the history of neuroscience.* Cambridge, MA: MIT Press.

Harvey, B. M., & Dumoulin, S. O. (2016). Visual motion transforms visual space representations similarly throughout the human visual hierarchy. *Neuroimage*, 127, 173–185.

Kuzawa, C. W., Chugani, H. T., Grossman, L. I., Lipovich, L., Muzik, O., Hof, P. R., . . . Lange, N. (2014). Metabolic costs and evolutionary implications of human brain development. *Proceedings of the National Academy of Sciences, 111*(36), 13010–13015.

Lashley, K. (1950). In search of the engram. In *Society for experimental biology #4: Mechanisms in animal behavior.* New York: Cambridge University Press.

Lezak, M. D. (2004). *Neuropsychological assessment.* Oxford: Oxford University Press.

Liang, H., & Wang, H. (2017). Structure-function network mapping and its assessment via persistent homology. *PLoS Computational Biology, 13*(1), 1–19.

Luria, A. R. (1973). *The working brain: An introduction to neuropsychology* (Trans. B. Haigh). New York: Basic Books.

Monti, M. M., Schnakers, C., Korb, A. S., Bystritsky, A., & Vespa, P. M. (2016). Non-invasive ultrasonic thalamic stimulation in disorders of consciousness after severe brain injury: A first-in-man report. *Brain Stimulation, 9*(6), 940.

Pal, G., Persinger, V., Bernard, B., Ouyang, B., Goetz, C., & Metman, L. V. (2016). The Core Assessment Program for Surgical Interventional Therapies in Parkinson's Disease (CAPSIT-PD): Tolerability of preoperative neuropsychological testing for deep brain stimulation in Parkinson's disease. *Neurology, 86*(16 Supplement), P3–357.

Pang, E. W., & Snead III, O. C. (2016). From structure to circuits: The contribution of MEG connectivity studies to functional neurosurgery. *Frontiers in Neuroanatomy*, 10.

Racanello, A. M., Tomb, M. F., Algermissen, M., & Margolis, A. (2016). The nuts and bolts of pediatric neuropsychological assessment: What it measures and how it can be helpful in diagnosing and treating children with neurodevelopmental disorders. *Journal of the American Academy of Child & Adolescent Psychiatry, 55*(10), S351.

Teter, T. (2000, May). *Pierre-Paul Broca.* Retrieved from www.muskingum.edu.

van Andel, J., Thijs, R. D., de Weerd, A., Arends, J., & Leijten, F. (2016). Non-EEG based ambulatory seizure detection designed for home use: What is available and how will it influence epilepsy care? *Epilepsy & Behavior, 57*, 82–89.

Wheless, J. W., Castillo, E., Maggio, V., Kim, H. L., Breier, J. I., Simos, P. G., & Papanicolaou, A. C. (2004). Magnetoencephalography (MEG) and magnetic source imaging (MSI). *The Neurologist, 10*(3), 138–153.

Wu, J. Y., Sutherling, W. W., Koh, S., Salamon, N., Jonas, R., Yudovin, S., . . . Mathern, G. W. (2006). Magnetic source imaging localizes epileptogenic zone in children with tuberous sclerosis complex. *Neurology, 66*(8), 1270–1272.

Wyllie, E., Comair, Y. G., Kotagal, P., Bulacio, J., Bingaman, W., & Ruggieri, P. (1998). Seizure outcome after epilepsy surgery in children and adolescents. *Annals of Neurology, 44*(5), 740–748.

Yildirim, F. B., & Sarikcioglu, L. (2007). Marie Jean Pierre Flourens (1794–1867): An extraordinary scientist of his time. *Journal of Neurology, Neurosurgery & Psychiatry, 78*(8), 852.

Yuste, R. (2015). From the neuron doctrine to neural networks. *Nature Reviews Neuroscience, 16*(8), 487–497.

Zillmer, E. A., Spiers, M. V., & Culbertson, W. C. (2008). *Principles of neuropsychology*. Belmont, CA: Thomson Higher Education.

2

THE BRAIN'S FUNCTIONS AND STRUCTURES

Information about brain structures and functions can help explain how brain growth and neurological development contribute to many areas of development. Without a firm basic knowledge of the structures and functions of the nervous system and the brain, it is not possible to understand brain research or critically evaluate its implications for education, social services, parenting, or policy. This chapter is intended to change the reader's mental schema regarding the brain from "terra incognita" to "terra cognita" (unknown to known land), because the development of a meaningful mental schema of the brain is needed to assimilate current research findings on brain functioning. Scientists now have a relatively clear general picture of the basic components of the nervous system, the structures of the brain, and the role these components and structures play in human physical and mental development and functioning. Theorists also have proposed hypotheses about how the brain works, and made models or metaphors of its structure and functions that can help in constructing mental schema to use in translating brain research into meaningful educational and social service theory, policy making, and practice.

Theoretical Evolutionary Foundations of the Brain

One of the earlier models of brain structure in the twentieth century was proposed by a former US National Institute of Mental Health Brain and Behavior Lab Director, Paul MacLean (1982). He hypothesized that the human brain was "triune," with three structural levels that evolved separately over time. Theorists indicate that because human's ancient survival patterns are lodged in the most primitive of the three brains, the development of compassion, empathy, and concern for future humans required the most recent addition: the prefrontal lobes

(Caine & Caine, 1991). MacLean labeled the three levels of the triune brain *reptilian*, *mammalian*, and *neomammalian*. While more recent research calls into question some reported aspects of triune brain research and stresses instead the interactive nature of different areas of the brain, this model still has usefulness as a functional metaphor for understanding the evolutionary development of the brain. In MacLean's model, the brain stem, medulla, pons, and cerebellum, which are responsible for basic body survival functions (such as digestion, reproduction, circulation, breathing, and "fight or flight" responses), compose the *reptilian* brain (or the hindbrain). This was the earliest part of the brain to develop in humans, and may play the largest role in deceptive behavior as part of our ethics of security (Narvaez, 2008). MacLean's *mammalian* brain (or midbrain) is part of the limbic system, which houses humans' primary centers for emotion, locale memory, smell, food, and sex, which reside in connections between the amygdala and hippocampus. The process of connecting emotions to concepts or memorable situations is an important task for learners to undertake. The third level, *neomammalian* or forebrain, is called the cerebrum. MacLean, as well as researchers today, viewed this most recent brain area as being responsible for complex and higher mental thought processes, inhibition, abstraction, attention, and future planning. This area of the brain is the last part to develop fully during the lifespan, and it is essential for critical examination of the world and thoughtful action.

Brain Functions

The communication functions of the brain are carried out by the neurons, each of which is composed of a cell body, one axon (sending unit), and a number of dendrites (receiving units). Neurons are not attached to each other; rather, there are gaps between the axon and dendrites of each neuron, which are called synapses. Each neuron communicates through electrical impulses sent through the axon and dendrites and through chemical agents (neurotransmitters) that "jump the gap" at the synaptic site. There are over 100 neurotransmitters that are activated by the correct "fit" with certain receptor sites. Each class of neurotransmitters appears to be involved with particular categories of activation, such as memory or emotional arousal (Lezak, 1995; Friedman et al., 2013). The brain also contains blood vessels that nourish the neurons, thus enabling them to function. The brain tissues are extremely oxygen-dependent; thus, they rely greatly on the oxygen transmitted through the blood vessels (Powers, 1990). Although the brain weighs only about 3 pounds in adults (about 10% of an adult's total weight), it uses about 25% of the adult's blood supply. The neuronal communication system is shown in Figure 2.1.

At birth, infant brains contain about 100 billion energy-consuming neurons, each of which can produce up to 15,000 synapses when they are well-nourished and adequately stimulated. Nutrients, omega-3 fatty acids, docosahexaenoic acid (DHA), and selective minerals like iodine, iron, zinc, and copper are in high demand

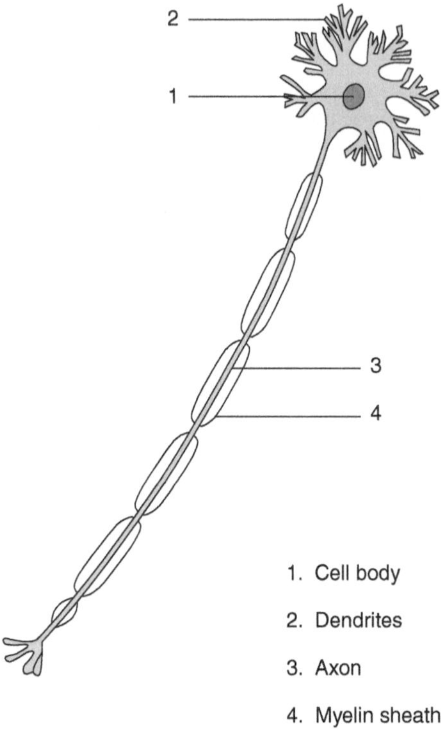

FIGURE 2.1 Brain Nervous System Components

by the infant brain (Cunnane & Crawford, 2014). From birth to age 3, synaptic density greatly increases and continues to increase, although not in an orderly pattern, during the early childhood years (Huttenlocher & Dabholkar, 1997). "This elaboration of neurons and increased synaptic potential constitutes the neural basis of learning, knowledge, ability, and skill" (Lezak, 1995, p. 47). These alterations in the brain's circuitry add to the brain's "long-term potentiation" for flexible and varied human behavior. Although some pruning occurs at earlier ages (Lichtman, 2001), that process increases by age 8 or 9 and synapses that have not been activated frequently begin to be eliminated or weakened. Current research focusing on developmental peaks in synaptogenesis and adult neurogenesis suggests that the brain employs complex learning mechanisms requiring generating new neurons, eliminating synapses, and maintaining portions of the newborn neural network (Bruel-Jungerman, Davis, & Laroche, 2007). These factors contribute to the overall plasticity and health of the human brain and are the most important influences on learning from infant to adult (see Zatorre, Fields, & Johansen-Berg, 2012, for an example of the plasticity of the brain in learning).

The messages sent by neurons are communicated among the structures of the brain and through the spinal cord to and from the nerves in the rest of the body. The brain and spinal cord together form the central nervous system (CNS). The supporting glia cells provide a fatty substance (myelin) that coats the axons, making message transmission faster and more efficient. Recently, research has indicated that one type of glia (astrocytes) may serve a number of other functions, such as supplying neurons with glucose, blocking toxic substances, and stimulating the generation of synapses (Netting, 2001). They also may store memory information and strengthen neural messages between neurons (Netting, 2001). Neurons from various structures communicate within the brain. Those concerned with processing emotions are in touch with those involved in rational decision-making, and both communicate with the autonomic system. Similarly, messages communicated to and from the brain to the body regulate behavior and thought. For example, the sensory and motor centers of the brain direct the muscles involved in bicycle riding, and when a rough pavement is encountered, the sensory and motor input from the arms and legs provide information to the brain so that it can signal changes in motor coordination. Although much brain research has been focused on identifying brain structures and determining which areas of the brain are involved in various processes (e.g., vision, hearing, movement, language, perception), more recent research has rejected an "isolated operations" perspective on cognition. Bressler and Menon (2010, p. 277) state, "the weight of evidence has now shifted in support of the view that cognition results from the dynamic interactions of distributed brain areas operating in large-scale networks" and they note that the structures of the brain are not independent processors but are part of a "conjoint function of brain areas working together as large-scale networks" (p. 277). The following description of brain structures should be viewed within this network framework.

Brain Structures

The brain is composed of the nerve cell bodies, the fibers (axons and dendrites), the glia (supporting and activating cells), and the blood vessels. There are also a series of open spaces (ventricles) through which cerebrospinal fluid flows. This fluid serves as a shock absorber and helps maintain the shape of the softer brain tissue. In general, the three major anatomical divisions of the brain (brain stem, limbic system, cerebrum) are successively more complex in organization (Goldberg, 1990; Friedman et al., 2013). Figure 2.2 shows the basic structures of the brain.

The Cerebral Cortex

The cortex has two hemispheres (right, left) and four lobes in each hemisphere. Each hemisphere contains white matter (axon, dendrites) and gray matter (cell bodies). The cortex has dense folds that in the adult brain, if stretched flat, would cover about 2.5 square feet, about the size of a chamois cloth. The bulges in the

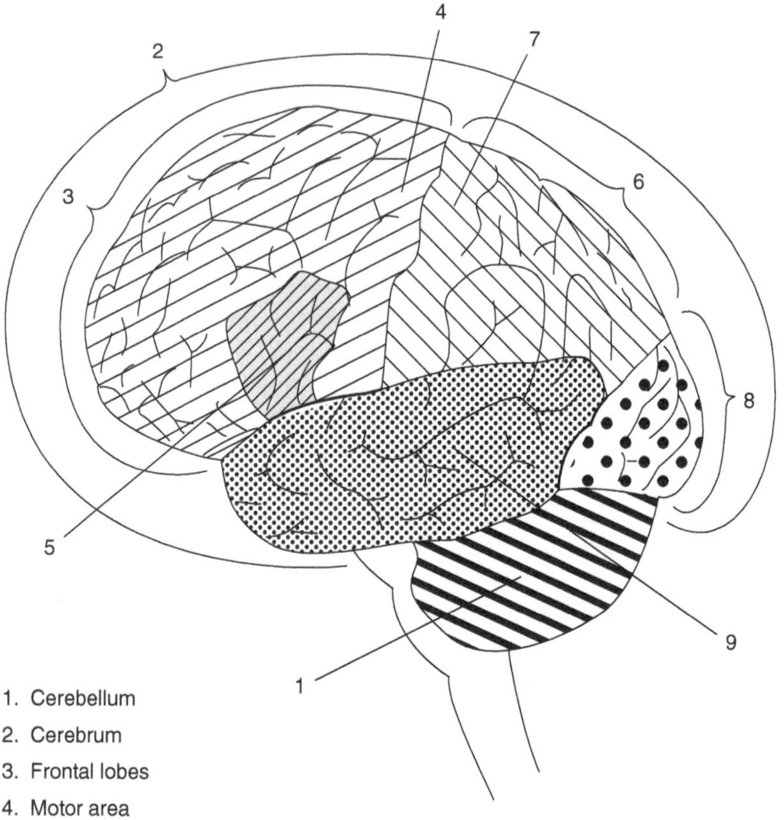

1. Cerebellum
2. Cerebrum
3. Frontal lobes
4. Motor area
5. Broca's area (language)
6. Parietal lobes
7. Sensory areas
8. Occipital lobes
9. Temporal lobes

FIGURE 2.2 Brain Areas

folds are called "gyri" and the indentations are called "sulci" or, if deep, "fissures." The four lobes in each hemisphere are called frontal, parietal, occipital, and temporal, and each has some distinctive functions, although specific behaviors are not totally localized. The top of the frontal lobe has the primary motor cortex and the mid-section holds an area having primary motor control of language (usually more pronounced in the dominant hemisphere). In the front (anterior) of the cortex is the primary site of functions such as initiative, drive, and the ability to control impulses, follow social rules, and perceive and reflect on actions. The somatosensory cortex, which primarily governs sensory processing, is located in the parietal lobe, and this lobe also has an area that controls the perception and interpretation of written language. Vision is located primarily in the occipital (back) lobe, and hearing and sound localization in the temporal (side) lobe, which also contains an area identified as vital for the interpretation of spoken language. While these areas are primary for certain functions, many other parts of the brain are involved in these functions. The white matter fibers (the axons) within each hemisphere project into subcortical areas, and some of these connect the two hemispheres. The connecting structure is called the corpus callosum. The deeper structures of the forebrain include the lateral ventricle (a C-shaped cavity), the basal ganglia, and the dorsal and ventral striatum, which are involved in intentional movement, the understanding of rewards, and some aspects of executive functioning. The cerebrospinal fluid (CSF), which is transported through the ventricles, is produced in this area.

While hemisphere specialization has been identified, there is much congruence between the left and right hemispheres. Often the dominant hemisphere (usually the left) is slightly larger, while certain areas in the right hemisphere may be larger (e.g., visuospatial). However, both the adult left/right brain and frontal lobe responses show little anatomic asymmetry, except in cases of abnormal development (Lezak, 1995; Song et al., 2015; Zhang et al., 2015). Lateralization (special functions) is most evident in the dominance of speech expression and sequential processing in the left hemisphere, and the ability to mediate complex, difficult-to-verbalize stimuli in the right hemisphere. The left hemisphere also may have superiority in processing detailed information and the right in processing large-scale or global concepts. Right-hemisphere capacities for comprehension and seeing relationships have been found, which are necessary for understanding alternative meanings and enjoying jokes (Lee et al., 2015; Lezak, 1995). Normal behavior, however, is a function of the whole brain, with both hemispheres contributing to most activities and emotions. Complex mental tasks such as reading or mathematics and effective storing and retrieving of memories need active engagement of both hemispheres.

The Limbic System

Embedded below the cerebral cortex is the area called the limbic system. It includes the thalamus, which relays and integrates information from sensory systems to the cortex; the hypothalamus, which is the master controller of the autonomic system; the hippocampus, which is involved in emotional reactions, understanding time, learning, and memory; and the amygdala, which perceives and interprets emotions, as well as receiving olfactory information. The thalamus also plays a role in arousing processing and response systems and regulating higher-level brain activity. The hypothalamus, through its control of the autonomic system, governs heart rate, body temperature, appetite and thirst, and sleep/waking cycles through both sympathetic (increasing physical responses) and parasympathetic (decreasing physical responses) processes. Through the pituitary gland, the hypothalamus also governs the endocrine system, which has glands located throughout the body that secrete hormones necessary for growth, sexual development, and other functions. Recent research has suggested that these structures are in close interaction with structures in the cortex, and thus they play a role in higher-order thinking as well. Figure 2.3 shows a diagram of this system.

The Brain Stem

In the brain stem, the cerebellum controls balance, posture, motor coordination, timing, and body space awareness (Breska & Ivry, 2016), and also has some involvement with attention, memory, learning, time perception, and touch (Goetz et al., 2014; Lezak, 1995). The medulla regulates functions such as breathing, swallowing, blood pressure, and reflex actions like sneezing. Through the medulla run the afferent (*to* higher-processing brain centers) and efferent (*from* higher-processing brain centers) fibers or axons that connect receptors and effectors in other parts of the body to the central nervous system (CNS). The pons links the cortex with the cerebellum and has a role in facial expression and eye movement. A network of interconnected nerve cell bodies and fibers form the reticular formation, which

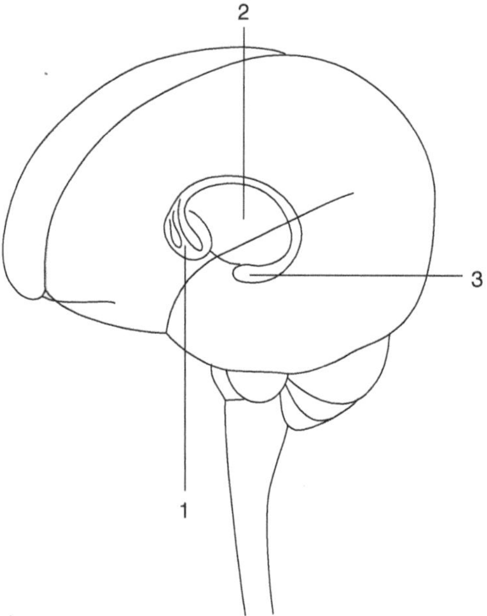

1. Hypothalamus
2. Thalamus
3. Hippocampus

FIGURE 2.3 Inner Brain (Limbic System) Components

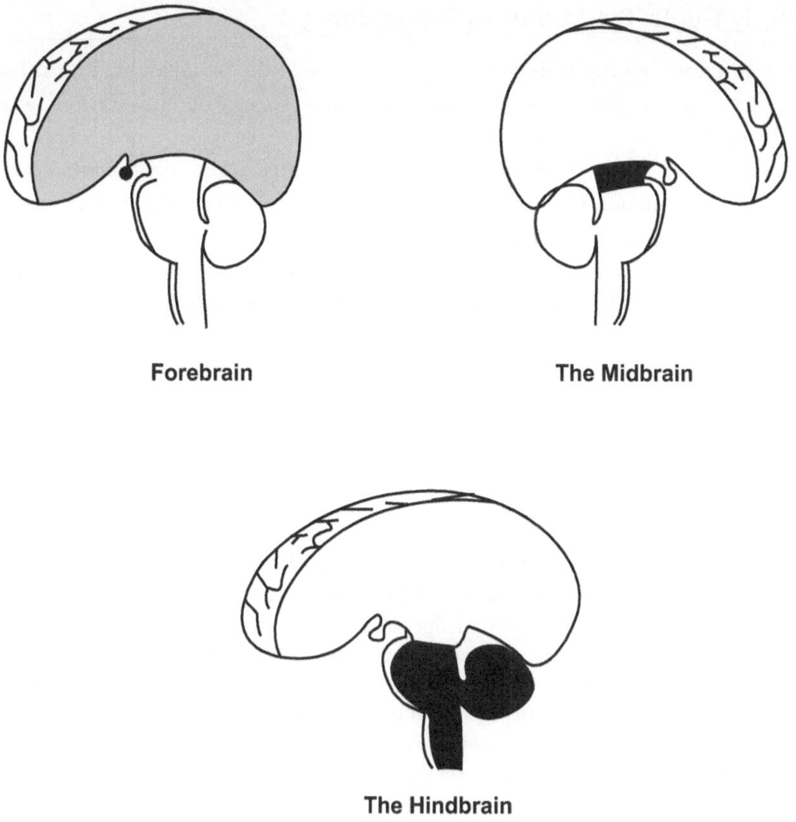

FIGURE 2.4 Brain Structural Components

holds the reticular activating system (RAS) responsible for controlling wakefulness and alertness. Figure 2.4 shows the relationship among the three brain areas. The Glossary has definitions of brain-related terms.

Brain Development

The brain structures and functions described in this chapter begin development during the prenatal period, show extensive growth during the infant and preschool-age periods, and continue to be modified and extended throughout the elementary, middle school, and adolescent years. There also are modifications that occur during adult life. Brain development is affected by many factors, some of which are genetic and some of which are environmental. Although there is still much to be studied and learned, a body of knowledge concerning brain development now exists and can provide a basis upon which parental, educational, and public policy decisions can be made (Richmond et al., 2016).

Study Guide/Questions for Discussion

- Without looking at diagrams, draw a picture of the brain, identifying at least six areas correctly. Draw and label the neurological communication network system.
- Prepare a short presentation on basic brain structures and functions. Give the presentation to an education class, teacher meeting, or parent event, and evaluate its effectiveness.
- Discuss societal implications of having accurate and extensive knowledge of brain functions and structures and how this knowledge could promote human brain development.
- List five points to use in a discussion with community individuals about potential misuse of brain images on products stating they are "brain-based" when research does not support that claim.

Bibliography

Breska, A., & Ivry, R. B. (2016). Taxonomies of timing: Where does the cerebellum fit in? *Current Opinion in Behavioral Sciences, 8*, 282–288.

Bressler, S. L., & Menon, V. (2010). Large-scale brain networks in cognition: Emerging methods and principles. *Trends in Cognitive Sciences, 14*(6), 277–290.

Bruel-Jungerman, E., Davis, S., & Laroche, S. (2007). Brain plasticity mechanisms and memory: a party of four. *The Neuroscientist, 13*(5), 492-505.

Caine, R. N., & Caine, G. (1991). *Making connections: Teaching and the human brain*. Alexandria, VA: Association for Supervision and Curriculum Development.

Coulson, S., & Wu, Y. C. (2005). Right hemisphere activation of joke-related information: An event-related brain potential study. *Journal of Cognitive Neuroscience, 17*(3), 494–506.

Cunnane, S. C., & Crawford, M. A. (2014). Energetic and nutritional constraints on infant brain development: Implications for brain expansion during human evolution. *Journal of Human Evolution*, 77, 88–98.

Federmeier, K. D., Wlotko, E. W., & Meyer, A. M. (2008). What's 'Right' in language comprehension: Event-related potentials reveal right hemisphere language capabilities. *Language and Linguistics Compass, 2*(1), 1–17.

Friedman, S. L., Klivington, K. A., & Peterson, R. W. (Eds.). (2013). *The brain, cognition, and education*. New York: Academic Press.

Goetz, M., Vesela, M., & Ptacek, R. (2014). Notes on the role of the cerebellum in ADHD. *Austin Journal of Psychiatry and Behavioral Science, 1*(3), 6.

Goldberg, S. (1990). *Clinical neuroanatomy made ridiculously simple*. Miami, FL: MedMaster, Inc.

Gross, C. G. (1998). *Brain, vison, memory: Tales in the history of neuroscience*. Cambridge, MA: MIT Press.

Huttenlocher, P. R., & Dabholkar, A. S. (1997). Regional differences in synaptogenesis in human cerebral cortex. *Journal of Comparative Neurology, 387*(2), 167–178.

Jones, W. H. S., & Withington, E. T. (1923). The sacred disease. *Hippocrates Works With English Translation, 2*, 127–183.

Lashley, K. (1950). In search of the engram. In *Society for experimental biology #4: Mechanisms in animal behavior*. New York: Cambridge University Press.

Lee, K. H., Mathews, P. J., Reeves, A. M., Choe, K. Y., Jami, S. A., Serrano, R. E., & Otis, T. S. (2015). Circuit mechanisms underlying motor memory formation in the cerebellum. *Neuron, 86*(2), 529–540.

Lezak, M. D. (1995). *Neuropsychological assessment* (3rd ed.). New York: Oxford.

Lichtman, J. W. (2001). Developmental neurobiology overview: Synapses, circuits, and plasticity. In D. B. Bailey, J. T. Bruer, F. J. Symons, & J. W. Lichtman (Eds.), *Critical thinking about critical periods* (pp. 27–42). Baltimore, MD: Paul H. Brookes.

Lindquist, K. A., & Barrett, L. F. (2012). A functional architecture of the human brain: Emerging insights from the science of emotion. *Trends in Cognitive Sciences, 16*(11), 533–540.

Luria, A. R. (1973). *The working brain: An introduction to neuropsychology* (Trans. B. Haigh). New York: Basic Books.

MacLean, P. D. (1982). On the origin and progressive evolution of the triune brain. In *Primate brain evolution* (pp. 291–316). New York: Springer.

Narvaez, D. (2008). Triune ethics: The neurobiological roots of our multiple moralities. *New Ideas in Psychology, 26*(1), 95–119.

Netting, J. (2001). Gray matters: Neurons get top billing but lesser-known brain cells also star. *Science News, 159*, 222–223.

Powers, W. J. (1990). Stroke. In A. L. Pearlman & R. C. Collins (Eds.), *Neurobiology of disease* (pp. 339–355). New York: Oxford University Press.

Richmond, S., Johnson, K. A., Seal, M. L., Allen, N. B., & Whittle, S. (2016). Review article: Development of brain networks and relevance of environmental and genetic factors: A systematic review. *Neuroscience and Biobehavioral Reviews, 71*, 215–239.

Song, J. W., Mitchell, P. D., Kolasinski, J., Grant, P. E., Galaburda, A. M., & Takahashi, E. (2015). Asymmetry of white matter pathways in developing human brains. *Cerebral Cortex, 25*(9), 2883–2893.

Wig, G. S., Schlaggar, B. L., & Petersen, S. E. (2011). Concepts and principles in the analysis of brain networks. *Annals of the New York Academy of Sciences, 1224*(1), 126–146.

Zatorre, R. J., Fields, R. D., & Johansen-Berg, H. (2012). Plasticity in gray and white: Neuroimaging changes in brain structure during learning. *Nature Neuroscience, 15*(4), 528–536.

Zhang, Y., Inder, T. E., Neil, J. J., Dierker, D. L., Alexopoulos, D., Anderson, P. J., & Van Essen, D. C. (2015). Cortical structural abnormalities in very preterm children at 7 years of age. *NeuroImage, 109*, 469–479.

3

PRENATAL BRAIN DEVELOPMENT AS A FOUNDATION FOR LEARNING

Case 1 Amala's Pregnancy Care

Amala (age 37) and her husband Jimmy (age 40) are expecting their first child and are busy planning for the baby's arrival. Both of their extended families are happy with this news and are eager for the baby's arrival. However, they are a little worried about Amala because she is at an older age for pregnancy. Also, Amala has had some health problems (incipient diabetes) and has been dieting in recent months to try to control this condition. She presently is working part-time as a nurse. She is following the advice of her doctor carefully, watching her diet and exercising regularly, and has given up her habit of occasional alcohol drinking when with friends. Jamal is attending both the doctor visits and the parenting classes with Amala, and he is making sure she takes her vitamins and other medications. At her last ultrasound session, they learned that the baby is a boy and that he is developing well, so that relieved some of their tension. They are beginning to read information about baby care and parenting but are also getting a lot of advice from friends and family. Unfortunately, the advice from their two families differs since they are from different cultures, and some of that advice conflicts with what they are learning in their pregnancy class and in their readings. They are beginning to think about what color they will paint the baby's room, what furniture to buy, and what to name him. Although Amala is excited and pleased about the baby's arrival, she has heard stories about pregnancy and delivery problems at her age and so, although she is happily awaiting her son's arrival, she also is very tense. Anecdotal stories from her friends and family have not always been helpful. However, she is determined to have a healthy baby and to be an excellent mother.

Case 2 Marge's Pregnancy Care

Marge (age 18) didn't expect to get pregnant and Larry (age 17) didn't expect to be a father while he was still in high school. Marge's parents were very unhappy when they heard this news, and they are very worried about the baby's healthy development, as well as whether they will be expected to care for the child after it is born. They are concerned because Marge has not changed her lifestyle yet (involving late hours and partying with friends), although her baby will be born in five months. Marge graduated from high school two months ago and is working part-time at Walmart. Larry has not seen Marge since she graduated, but she thinks it is because he and a pal are on a 100-mile bike ride that they had planned to do this summer. He hasn't been in contact with Marge though, and Marge is now thinking that he is not showing appropriate interest in the fact that she is having his baby. She is not sure if he plans to return to finish his last year of high school or whether he will take on any parenting responsibilities. Marge has stopped her occasional marijuana use but she hasn't been to a doctor regularly yet. At first, she acted as though her developing child did not exist. For example, she didn't tell her parents about the pregnancy until she started to look "fat." Her parents are nagging her about taking better care of herself, but she is still going out with friends most weekends. Marge had planned to take some courses at the local community college after she graduated from high school, but now she is not sure what she will do as her mother has said she is not going to be a full-time "babysitter." In fact, Marge's parents have suggested that it would be best if she agreed that the baby should be adopted. They think they know a family who might be interested.

Review of Prenatal Brain Development

In humans, about 60% of all genes are dedicated to brain development (Shore, 1997; Siegel, 2015), and during the prenatal period, the basic structures of the brain and neuronal network form. According to Corn and Bishop (2010), human brain development begins with "only a few undifferentiated cells" but these cells "set the stage for the construction of the nervous system that continues throughout embryonic, fetal, and postnatal life" (p. 1). Shortly after conception, the brain begins to develop from the neural tube, and the developmental direction is "from the neck up," beginning with the brain stem and ending with the cortex. Because most complex types of human behaviors are not genetically programmed, fetal brain development involves the generation of many more neurons than will eventually be needed. The neurons begin dividing and multiplying and the axons begin forming synaptic connections from the first few weeks of the prenatal period, although most neurons are generated during the second trimester (12 to 20 weeks). This is a "critical period" of prenatal development, because during this time period, the neurons begin to migrate from the lateral ventricle toward the skull, and they form layers of neurons, each built on top of earlier ones. According to Bielas et al. (2004), "Neuronal migration is a hallmark of cerebral cortical development" and it is "a highly choreographed process" (p. 149). The cortical cell migration, in which the neurons that will form the cortex develop in its deepest layers and travel up "cortical ladders" composed of glial cells to form the upper sections of the cortex, is a vital part of healthy brain development. As the cells proceed up these ladders, they encounter genes that define their purpose and final location. The process works from the bottom up; that is, the first migrating cells stop at a lower level and each wave of cells goes above the existing levels to a higher level. By the mid-gestation period, many neurons are involved in the migration process, forming the structures of the cerebral cortex (Rakic, 1995). Although Rakic hypothesized about the basic processes earlier, only recently have some of the genes underlying these functions been identified. For example, Bielas et al. (2004) have reported that the microtubule cytoskeleton appears to be important in the proper positioning of neurons within the cortex and in determining the rate at which neurons move. This period is especially important for the formation of higher brain centers, and thus problematic prenatal environments can have deleterious effects on cortical development.

The normally developing fetus begins to show motor and sensory activity very early (about seven weeks after gestation), and researchers have hypothesized that this activity aids early brain development (Hofer, 1988). Other brain areas that begin development early in fetal life are the somatosensory system (touch, pain, and temperature sensitivity); the vestibular system (balance and motion); and the visual, auditory, olfactory, and gustatory senses. An area (Wernicke) that involves the capacity for understanding language, which is located between the temporal and parietal lobes (planum temporale), begins to grow larger on the left side of the brain. EEG measures of preterm infants show that by 30 weeks, the two hemispheres of the brain already respond differently to language, with the left hemisphere being specialized for this activity. Memory also begins to show basic brain configurations in the fetal period. The building of the higher brain centers continues throughout pregnancy, and at birth the infant's neurons number about 100 billion. Although there is now evidence that some neuronal generation occurs after birth, the prenatal period is the primary period for neuronal structural growth.

Corn and Bishop (2010) have described some assessment methods used to help physicians understand how well the fetus is developing. For example, ultrasonography is used to chart the developmental progress of the fetus, and risk conditions can begin to be assessed by the first trimester. Blood tests are used if an abnormal ultrasound occurs or if the pregnancy is "high risk." High-risk conditions include maternal age over 35, family history of birth defects, and a previous child with birth defects. Amniocentesis, which involves gaining a sample of amniotic fluid, is conducted in special circumstances of high-risk pregnancy concern.

Impact of Prenatal Genetic/Environmental Interaction

Because brain research has clearly indicated that the prenatal environment affects optimum brain development, one of the first implications of this research is that of "do no harm" (Shore, 1997). It is essential that professionals communicate the need for all women to get early prenatal care. Prenatal influences on brain development include genetic factors (physiology of egg and sperm; genetic transmission, errors, and mutations) and environmental factors (intrauterine environment, maternal illness, maternal stress and self-care behaviors, maternal use of harmful substances). Interactions between genetic and environmental factors begin shortly after conception. Many studies report that prenatal malnourishment, exposure to teratogens (substances such as radiation, lead, nicotine, alcohol, and cocaine), and maternal illness and/or maternal stress can negatively affect specific aspects of early brain development, depending on the time period in which they occur. Specific nutritional deficiencies can be crucial at early stages; for example, a deficiency of folic acid in the first weeks of pregnancy may affect neural tube closure, resulting in spina bifida (Honein et al., 2001). Also, maternal stress has been linked to effects on limbic system development in children. Stress-triggered release of hormones (e.g., corticosteroids, catecholamine) from the hypothalamus-pituitary system may restrict blood flow and interfere with other aspects of brain development. Researchers have found that maternal smoking also negatively affects birth weight and is associated with lower scholastic achievement in children. They recommend programs to help pregnant women curb smoking because that would provide health benefits to both mother and offspring (Agrawal et al., 2010).

If teratogenic substances such as cocaine or alcohol are absorbed at the time cell migration is occurring, some of these cells may die and others may not reach the location for which they were destined. Such teratogens at early stages in fetal development may result in physical deformities, and at later stages may interfere with the production of synapses. Exposure to alcohol prenatally may distort this migration process so much that the result is fetal alcohol syndrome, which affects cognition and emotions. Ornoy and Ergaz (2010) have reported that high and repeated alcohol consumption may result in prenatal and postnatal growth deficiencies, craniofacial dysmorphic features, mental retardation, behavioral changes, and other anomalies, and they state that even moderate but repetitive alcohol use, including occasional binge drinking, may affect child intelligence, growth, and behavior. Heavy exposure to alcohol resulting in abnormal cortical thickness may be related to child behavior issues at later age periods (Sowell et al., 2008). Illnesses such as influenza also may interfere with the migration process and result in cognitive and emotional impairments. Researchers believe that some neurological disorders such as epilepsy may result from a distortion in the process of migration (Rakic, Bourgeois, & Goldman-Rakic, 1994). Recently the current outbreak of microcephaly reported in the Americas has brought attention to the possible deleterious effects that the Zika virus may have on fetal brain development because it interferes with this "brain building" process. Research is beginning to show that, in addition to microcephaly, there may be a link between the Zika virus infection and hydrops fetalis, fetal demise, and other fetal development problems (Adibi et al., 2016; Sarno et al., 2016).

General nutritional deficiencies may be more critical at later stages, resulting in infants with low birth weight and smaller head size. Morse (2012) has reported that if supplements such as docosahexaenoic acid (DHA), folic acid, vitamin D, and iodine can be given prenatally and during the nursing period, these supplements can prolong high-risk pregnancies; increase birth weight, head circumference, and birth length; and enhance visual acuity, hand-eye coordination, attention, problem-solving, and information processing. Thus, she recommends that supplementation within recommended guidelines for women with dietary deficiencies may improve infant brain and central nervous system functioning and overall brain development.

The prevalence of childhood cognitive and behavioral deficits is even more common in surviving preterm infants (Marlow et al., 2005; Delobel-Ayoub et al., 2009). Ball and colleagues (2012) have concluded that preterm infants often show altered brain structure patterns related to disruption of thalamocortical development (i.e., cerebral gray and white matter abnormalities). Studies focused on the effects of very low birth weight (under 750 grams) indicate that such infants have a higher incidence of neurological and mental impairments (Eliot, 1999; Marlow et al., 2005), and the effects may cause problems even at elementary and middle-school age, with more low birth weight children evidencing developmental, behavioral, and learning problems (Anderson & Doyle, 2003, Delobel-Avoub et al., 2009; Taylor et al., 2000).

Although most prenatal research has focused on negative impacts of poor fetal environments, research on some aspects of the prenatal environment show that some positive learning may occur prenatally. For example, research has shown that neonates attend more to the sound of their mothers' voices than to other voices, which implies that they have learned to recognize that voice in utero, and this recognition may be paired with early maternal facial recognition as well (Sai, 2005). Of course, maternal efforts to have good nutrition and to avoid teratogenic substances also are positive influences on growth and development (Fowles, 2004). More research focused on ways to improve prenatal care for groups who do not presently have access to such care has been advocated by numerous groups.

Newborn Brains

The infant arrives in the world with a set of basic reflexes that are involuntary, automatic, and complex but also stereotypical, and these are mediated through the brain stem and spinal cord (Bergen & Woodin, 2011). These reflexes may serve as "defensive" mechanisms initially that allow the infant to survive outside the womb. Reflexive movements gradually diminish during the first six months of life; however, some reflexive movements are present throughout life.

Recently, there has been interest in studying the neurodevelopment of newborns and very young infants to determine the characteristics of brain development that newborns bring into the world. Two methods have been used to study the neonate brain. Techniques for using magnetic resonance imaging (MRI) with newborns have been developed during the past ten to twelve years (see Richards & Xie, 2015, for details), and this method has provided information about neurostructural development of infants as young as 2 weeks (see Almli, Rivkin, & McKinstray, 2007), resulting in a "Neurodevelopmental MRI Database" (Richards & Xie, 2015, p. 9). The earliest age scans show little brain myelination, but by 3 months, "the posterior limb of the internal capsule is fully myelinated" (p. 14) and myelination proceeds rapidly during early childhood. The most rapid synaptic growth is between birth and 6 years, and the most rapid pruning is between 6 years and 14 years. Figure 3.1 shows synaptic development at birth, 6 years, and 14 years.

Newborns' brain activity also has been studied by measuring brain waves (EEG) and event-related potentials (ERP), which show brain wave patterns that occur when various stimuli are presented. For example, Winkler et al. (2009)

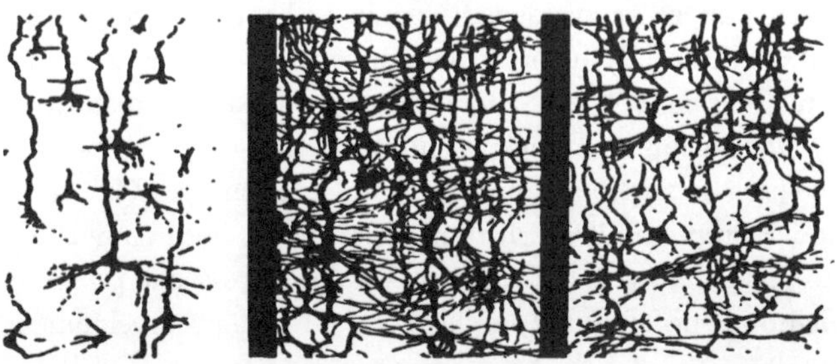

FIGURE 3.1 Synaptic Density From Birth to Adolescence

examined whether sleeping newborns would react to differences in rhythmic beats. They measured ERP responses to sound beat differences by giving varied sound sequences and found that when the beat of a rhythmic sound is violated, the newborn brain detects this violation. They concluded that there is auditory learning in the womb and the newborn's auditory system already has the capability of being sensitive to rhythmic cycles. Fifer et al. (2010) investigated whether newborn infants can learn from experiences by recording neonate electroencephalogram (EEG) activity during an eye-movement conditioning experiment in which a tone was followed by a puff of air to the infant's eye. The sleeping newborns showed an EEG slow wave after training that the experimenters hypothesized reflected memory updating. The effects of preterm infants' gestational age on how the brain processes information also has been studied. Bisiacchia, Mentoa, and Supplejb (2009) compared the difference in auditory ERPs of extremely low (23–29 weeks) and low (30–34 weeks) gestational-age newborns and concluded that their gestational age did have an influence on early cortical functioning. There may be long-term implications of newborn brain capabilities on children's later development. For example, Guttorm et al. (2010) found that newborn measures of brain activity predicted later potential for dyslexia. During the next decade, knowledge of newborn infants' emotional and cognitive abilities will be greatly enhanced by these neuropsychological research techniques.

Suggestions for Fostering Optimal Prenatal Brain Development

In spite of evidence that the prenatal environment is vitally important for good brain development, there are children born every day throughout the world who do not have an optimum start in life because of poor prenatal conditions. Some conditions are severe (e.g., mothers in starvation situations or with diseases contracted during pregnancy), but others are amenable to improvement (e.g., mothers with exposure to smoking, alcohol or other drugs, or with unhealthy diets). Unfortunately, evidence is clear that poor prenatal care may result in problematic issues related to health, disabilities, or behaviors in childhood or even at later ages. Many problems might be avoided if women had more attention, support, and information about healthy prenatal environments that promote optimum brain development. Recent concern about disproportionate prematurity rates and deaths of young infants from diverse and minority groups has been noted, and nation-wide programs are beginning to address this issue (see Centers for Disease Control and Prevention, 2002). It is imperative that both familial and societal attention to good prenatal and early infant care be increased to promote excellent prenatal environments and thus excellent fetal and infant development. Suggestions include:

For Families

- It is vital that family members support pregnant women's good health and nutritional practices and make sure that they receive good prenatal medical care. Relevant family members should participate in all aspects of that care in positive ways.
- Family environments lacking in positive social-emotional elements or promoting high levels of stress should be avoided by pregnant women.
- Because poverty has been shown to accompany instances of poor brain development, all families with infants and young children should have access to good nutrition, early care, and minimization or removal of teratogens within their environment.
- If pregnant women are smoking or using drugs, alcohol, or other harmful substances, outreach programs should assist them in conquering those addictions during the pregnancy period.

For Educarers and Educators

- Education about the importance of the prenatal period for brain development should be given in high school to both male and female students. Parent educators should work with potential parents to help them learn to provide healthy, safe, nurturing environments for their expected children and to gain access to needed environmental supports.
- Educators should encourage potential parents and pregnant women who have habits that will make fetal development more problematic to put aside those habits during the prenatal period (and beyond).

For Community Partners and Policy Makers

- Community partners should provide access to good prenatal care at reasonable cost in their communities, and parents who need transportation to such facilities should gain that assistance.
- Community partners should provide information about care assistance that is readily available to pregnant population groups who might not have access to such care.
- Community support for planning of pregnancies should be available so that pregnancy occurs when such support is available.
- Monitoring of low birth weight and premature infants should be ongoing, and efforts to reduce deaths of minority and low-income infants should be a focus of efforts.
- Funding for programs that support pregnancy planning, excellent prenatal care, and reduced infant mortality should be available in every community.

- Information on long-term societal effects of the lack of supports for healthy fetal development should be available to lawmakers during policy and funding decision- making.
- International programs that support pregnancy planning and pregnancy health care should be supported.

Case 3 Jenine's Pregnancy Care

Jenine (age 24) has just had a pregnancy test and found out that she is pregnant again. She is a single parent who already has a child of 2 and a child of 4. When her first two children were born, she was in a live-in relationship with Ray, the father of the 2-year-old. However, she has been in a relationship with Harley since then, and he is the father of this latest baby. She presently has no visible support system because the father of this latest child is facing a prison sentence for suspected child abuse related to Jenine's 2-year-old. Her parents live in another state and rarely visit her. She is presently on welfare and receiving food stamps. Jenine has sporadically tried to be a good parent to her children and has taken advantage of other services provided in her county, such as Women, Infants, Children (WIC). She also enrolled her 4-year-old in Head Start, but his attendance has been erratic. For a while, the 2-year-old was getting home-based infant visits, but that worker is the one who reported suspected abuse by her latest male companion, so Janine has not wanted contact with the worker again. Because of problems with her other children, the social services department has been involved in monitoring the children's welfare and they are discussing whether the children should continue to remain in her custody. Janine has had a history of depression and alcoholism. She is receiving counseling related to her alcohol abuse because it could affect the development of her fetus. The social worker does not see a healthy prognosis in the current situation, but is trying hard to convince Janine to stop behaviors that may be harmful in her latest pregnancy.

Case 4 Baby Elijah's Premature Arrival

Deloise was surprised about the news of her pregnancy, but she was happy about it because she was in a committed relationship with

Kenny and they both adjusted to the news well. For a long time, however, she did not really think about changing her lifestyle to accommodate a baby as she was a university student studying social work and hoping to get her license to practice; thus, her schedule was very demanding. Kenny often was not there to remind her to take it easy since, as a long-distance truck driver, he is gone for extended periods of time. When Deloise went to the doctor for her six-month checkup, the doctor expressed some concerns that the baby did not weigh as much as might be expected, and she urged Deloise to eat a better diet and to rest more. Shortly after that, Deloise began to have occasional pain, which at first she ignored but finally could not ignore; and when she reported that to the doctor, she was advised to have bed rest in order to avoid a premature delivery. Since the college term was ending in three weeks, she thought that she could wait that long to begin a less intense schedule, even though she did have some occasional pain. Fortunately, Kenny arrived home at the end of the second of those weeks, and he insisted that Deloise go to the hospital because the pains were getting stronger. After only a few hours at the hospital, Deloise gave birth to a son, Elijah, whose birth weight was only 720 grams. He was immediately taken to neonatal intensive care and it was expected that, although he would probably survive, his hospital stay would be extended. The prognosis for his development is presently unclear. Deloise now blames herself for her baby's problems, although the doctor has assured her that there are many factors that result in premature birth, and the cause of this happening is not clear. She is spending much of her summer time with the baby at the hospital, however, as the staff encourages mothers to be with their premature infants as much as possible.

Study Guide/Questions for Discussion

- Review the information on prenatal brain development and draw a timeline showing the course of that development over the nine months of pregnancy. Indicate what crucial types of development occur at various stages in the pregnancy.
- Compare issues that Amala, Marge, Jenine, and Deloise faced in ensuring that the prenatal environment was optimal for their infants. Discuss what they should do to ensure their infants' development will be supported. List what they have in common and what is different about the problems they must solve. Give suggestions for health and caregiving services they could access

to foster healthy brain development during the prenatal period and after the infant's birth.

- Compare the issues that a premature baby might face with those of a full-term infant. What are important concerns for the premature child and what supports are needed for their parents?
- Describe how you would evaluate the life chances of children who do not receive good prenatal care. What issues could affect their prenatal brain development and subsequent life course?
- Using information in this chapter, plan a presentation pointing out the need for services and/or funding of pregnancy planning and prenatal care for women in your community.
- Discuss ways that families, parent educators, community, and policy makers can work together to ensure healthy brain development during the fetal period for all children.
- Identify societal implications of having babies born who have not had good prenatal and after-birth care, and discuss the impact of poor care on communities, nations, and the world.

Bibliography

Adibi, J. J., Marques, E. T., Cartus, A., & Beigi, R. H. (2016). Teratogenic effects of the Zika virus and the role of the placenta. *The Lancet, 387*(10027), 1587–1590.

Agrawal, A., Scherrer, J. F., Grant, J. D., Sartor, C. E., Pergadia, M. L., Duncan, A. E., . . . Xian, H. (2010). The effects of maternal smoking during pregnancy on offspring outcomes. *Preventive Medicine, 50*(1), 13–18.

Almli, C. R., Rivkin, M. J., & McKinstray, R. C. (2007). The NIH MRI study of normal brain development (objective-2): Newborns, infant, toddlers, and preschoolers. *Neuro-Image, 35*(1), 308–325.

Anderson, P., Doyle, L. W., & Victorian Infant Collaborative Study Group. (2003). Neurobehavioral outcomes of school-age children born extremely low birth weight or very preterm in the 1990s. *JAMA, 289*(24), 3264–3272.

Ball, G., Boardman, J. P., Rueckert, D., Aljabar, P., Arichi, T., Merchant, N., Gousias, I. S., Edwards, A. D., & Counsell, S. J. (2012). The effect of preterm birth on thalamic and cortical development. *Cerebral Cortex, 22*(5), 1016–1024. doi:10.1093/cercor/bhr176.

Bergen, D., & Woodin, M. (2011). Neuropsychological development of newborns, infants, and toddlers. In A. S. Davis (Ed.), *Handbook of pediatric neuropsychology* (pp. 15–30). New York: Springer.

Bielas, S., Higginbotham, H., Koizumi, H., Tanaka, T., & Gleeson, J. G. (2004). Cortical neuronal migration mutants suggest separate but intersecting pathways. *Annual Review of Cell and Developmental Biology, 20*, 593–618.

Bisiacchia, P. S., Mentoa, G., & Supplejb, A. (2009). Cortical auditory processing in preterm newborns: An ERP study. *Biological Psychology, 82*(2), 176–185.

Centers for Disease Control and Prevention (CDC). (2002). Infant mortality and low birth weight among black and white infants—United States, 1980–2000. *MMWR. Morbidity and Mortality Weekly Report, 51*(27), 589.

Corn, H. J. M., & Bishop, D. L. (2010). Intrauterine development of the central nervous system. In A. S. Davis (Ed.), *Handbook of pediatric neuropsychology* (pp. 1–14). New York: Springer Publishing.

Delobel-Ayoub, M., Arnaud, C., White-Koning, M., Casper, C., Pierrat, V., Garel, M., . . . Kaminski, M. (2009). Behavioral problems and cognitive performance at 5 years of age after very preterm birth: The EPIPAGE Study. *Pediatrics, 123*(6), 1485–1492.

Eliot, L. (1999). *What's going on in there: How the brain and mind develop in the first five years of life*. New York: Bantam.

Fifer, W. P., Byrd, D. L., Kaku, M., Eigsti, I., Isler, J. R., Grose-Fifer, J., Tarullo, A. R., & Balsam, P. D. (2010). Newborn infants learn during sleep. *Proceedings of the National Academy of Sciences, 107*(22), 10320–10323.

Fowles, E. R. (2004). Prenatal nutrition and birth outcomes. *Journal of Obstetric, Gynecologic, & Neonatal Nursing, 33*(6), 809–822.

Guttorm, T. K., Leppanen, P. H., & Dawson, M. (2010). Newborn event-related potentials predict poorer pre-reading skills in children at risk for dyslexia. *Journal of Disability, 43*(5), 391–401.

Hofer, M. A. (1988). On the nature and function of prenatal behavior. In W. Smotherman & J. S. Robinson (Eds.), *Behavior of the fetus* (pp. 3–18). Caldwell, NJ: Telford.

Honein, M. A., Paulozzi, L. J., Mathews, T. J., Erickson, J. D., & Wong, L. Y. C. (2001). Impact of folic acid fortification of the US food supply on the occurrence of neural tube defects. *JAMA, 285*(23), 2981–2986.

Marlow, N., Wolke, D., Bracewell, M. A., & Samara, M. (2005). Neurologic and developmental disability at six years of age after extremely preterm birth. *New England Journal of Medicine, 352*(1), 9–19.

Morse, N. L. (2012). Benefits of docosahexaenoic acid, folic acid, vitamin D, and iodine on foetal and infant brain development and function following maternal supplementation during pregnancy and lactation. *Neurophysiologie Clinique/Clinical Neurophysiology, 42*, 35–41. doi:10.1016/j.neucli.2011.08.005.

Ornoy, A., & Ergaz, Z. (2010). Alcohol abuse in pregnant women: Effects on the fetus and newborn, mode of action and maternal treatment. *International Journal of Environmental Research and Public Health*, 7(2), 364–379.

Rakic, P. (1995). Corticogenesis in human and nonhuman primates. In M. S. Gazzaniga (Ed.), *The cognitive neurosciences* (pp. 127–145). Cambridge, MA: MIT Press.

Rakic, P., Bourgeois, J. P., & Goldman-Rakic, P. S. (1994). Synaptic development of the cerebral cortex: Implications for learning, memory, and mental illness. *Progress in Brain Research, 102*, 227–243.

Richards, J. E., & Xie, W. (2015). Chapter one—Brains for all the ages: Structural neurodevelopment in infants and children from a life-span perspective. *Advances in Child Development and Behavior, 48*, 1–52. Elsevier. doi:10.1016/bs.acdb.2014.11.001. Epub February 7, 2015.

Sai, F. Z. (2005). The role of the mother's voice in developing mother's face preference: Evidence for intermodal perception at birth. *Infant and Child Development, 14*(1), 29–50.

Sarno, M., Sacramento, G. A., Khouri, R., do Rosário, M. S., Costa, F., Archanjo, G., Santos, L. A., Nery, Jr., N., Vasilakis, N., Ko, A. I., de Almeida, A. R. P., & da Saúde da Bahia, E. (2016). Zika virus infection and stillbirths: A case of hydrops fetalis, hydranencephaly and fetal demise. *PLOS Neglected Tropical Diseases*. doi:10.1371/journal.pntd.0004517.

Shore, R. (1997). *Rethinking the brain: New insights into early development*. New York: Families and Work Institute.

Siegel, D. J. (2015). *The developing mind: How relationships and the brain interact to shape who we are*. New York: Guilford Publications.
Sowell, E. R., Mattson, S. N., Kan, E., Thompson, P. M., Riley, E. P., & Toga, A. W. (2008). Abnormal cortical thickness and brain–behavior correlation patterns in individuals with heavy prenatal alcohol exposure. *Cerebral Cortex, 18*(1), 136–144.
Taylor, H. G., Klein, N., Minich, N. M., & Hack, M. (2000). Middle-school-age outcomes in children with very low birthweight. *Child Development, 71*(6), 1495–1511.
Taylor, M. J., Khan, S. C., & Malone, M. A. (1999). Parallel and serial attentional processes: A developmental ERP study. *Developmental Neuropsychology, 15*(3), 351–358.
Winkler, I., Háden, G. P., Lading, O., Sziller, I., & Horning, H. (2009). Newborn infants detect the beat in music. *Proceedings of the National Academy of Sciences, 106*(7), 2468–2471.

4

BRAIN DEVELOPMENT AND LEARNING IN THE INFANT AND TODDLER YEARS

Case 1 Brent at 8 months

Brent weighed 7 pounds 2 ounces at birth and was 19 inches long, which is in the range of "typical" birth weight and length, and his development has followed an expected schedule. Brent's mother says he was an "easy" baby right from his birth. He adjusted to a regular feeding routine and by 3 months was sleeping through the night. He showed a "social smile" at 4 months, vocalized while manipulating the toys on his jumper seat, and attended to music and "baby" videos as he grew older. At 8 months, he is still good-natured and mostly cooperative, but also is becoming "strong-willed" according to parental reports. He was breast-fed until 6 months and is now bottle fed. He does not drink from a cup but can feed himself "finger food" such as cereal pieces and crackers. He sat up at 6 months and now crawls effectively, looks for toys when he drops them, and babbles various sounds, such as "baba." He is not yet standing alone, but he stands briefly, holding onto the sofa, if his father props him there. Brent's temperament continues to be calm and he has a relatively long attention span with toys—shaking keys, spinning dials, pressing buttons—and he looks briefly at books. He plays "peek-a-boo" with his parents but not with strangers. He is attached to his parents but does go willingly to the child care program he attends two days a week. The educarer there reports that Brent is attentive to other children's actions and is beginning to interact with them, although his usual behavior is watching for a long time before acting. Both his parents and the educarer would characterize him as having an "easy" temperament but as being "slow to warm up."

Case 2 Dana at Toddler Age

At 18 months, Dana is a dynamo of activity. She has been a healthy child and, as an infant, she enjoyed physical play and rhythmic motions more than lying quietly in her crib or sitting in her infant seat. She crawled early and started to walk at 11 months. Although she was compliant in feedings when she was younger, she is now a "picky eater" according to her mother. She can feed herself but has little patience for sitting in her high chair once she has finished eating. Dana has many interests, including "dancing" to music, climbing steps, and playing with the remote control on the television. She has begun to look at the apps on her mother's phone and has a few that she will play with for a short time. Dana is interested in anything that makes a noise, has motion, or provides many features to explore. She also likes to poke into kitchen cabinets, pulling apart and restacking pans and dishes. She is beginning to engage in pretend activities such as "feeding" a doll. At her child care center, she often attempts to replicate activities of the slightly older children in the group. She understands directions and will follow them when she is "in the mood." She also communicates her needs and wishes and remarks on events in "holophrastic" sentences such as "gookie, gookie" (for requesting a cookie) and commenting on events such as "daddy go car." She scribbles with crayons and sings versions of a few songs. Sometimes she has small tantrums when she does not immediately get her wishes met, but she usually follows directions and she has a good memory for routine activities. If the routine is changed, she sometimes gets upset. Her parents are amazed at how quickly Dana learns new behaviors—even ones that she observes that they would prefer she not exhibit. They say that every day she seems to have learned something new.

Review of Brain Development During the Infant Year

When a baby is born, most of the neurons that the child will have throughout life are already present, but the synaptic connections among neurons are not extensive. Thus, human brain development is highly affected by the environments with which the child interacts during the first three years of life. The growth in size and weight of the brain is caused by increases in the size of the neurons, greater dendritic connections, initial myelination of axons, and increases in glial cell size and number. Although the brain weighs only about 1 pound at birth, by age 1 it has increased in weight to about 2 pounds. Usually the first growth spurt happens during the age 3- to 4-month period. The amount of energy used by the brain changes as various parts develop, with the sensorimotor areas of the cortex (related to reflexive behaviors) being most active at first. By 2 or 3 months, activity becomes greater in the parietal, temporal, and primary visual cortex, basal ganglia, and cerebellar hemispheres (Bergen & Woodin, 2011). Some activities most enjoyed by infants during this age period, such as being touched, reaching for and touching people and objects, looking, tasting, and manipulating objects, and being bounced, swung, or lifted, are all relevant experiences that contribute to their coordination of voluntary movement and the further development of these brain areas. One common characteristic of infants is their ability to "eye gaze" as they look into the faces of other humans. In fact, this behavior is so characteristic that there is now research indicating that a lack of such eye gaze may be an early indicator of autism (Elsabbagh et al., 2012).

The frontal cortex areas of the brain begin to be active at about 6 months, and by 8 months there is a notable increase in activity in the frontal lobe, corresponding to higher infant cognitive functioning. By about 9 months, greater infant motor control enables them to interact meaningfully with objects and people in their environment, begin to understand language and express sounds used in that language, and to learn through imitating the actions of others. Infants of 6 months can discriminate and categorize phonemes (the smallest units of sounds we use in speech) from every language, but by 1 year they have learned to focus distinctly on phonemes from their native language (Kiester, 2001). By age 1, the dorsal and medial frontal regions show greater activity, and the metabolic activity of the cortex is similar to the activity of adult brains. Infants can express emotion at an early age because the amygdala, part of the limbic system, is well formed at birth; however, the limbic cortex, where emotions are recognized or "felt," matures during the 6- to 18-month period. The development of the medial frontal lobe is evidenced by the expression of infant attachment to caregivers and by stranger anxiety. Another social development, infant imitation of observed actions of others, appears to be related to the activation of "mirror neurons" located in the parietal and frontal lobe (Coude et al., 2016; Rizzolatti & Craighero, 2004). This phenomenon seems to help the child both imitate and understand the actions of others.

Studies of brain wave interactions show developmental changes during an infant's first year. For example, 4- and 5-month-old infants exposed to two rhythmic language conditions showed differences in brain waves with the two conditions, but by 5 months the infants' brain wave patterns were similar to those of adult subjects. The 5-month-old infants showed a pattern indicating that they could discriminate between the "correct" pronunciation and "incorrect" pronunciation of the stimuli (Weber et al., 2004). Also, infants age 6 to 9 and 10 to 12 months exposed to Spanish, English, and combined stimuli sounds did not show discrimination of the stimuli at the younger age, but at the older age they did show significant differences in peak amplitude between the various stimuli, reflecting better phoneme discrimination (Garcia-Sierra et al., 2011). A longitudinal study by Bell and Wolfe (2007) examined how infants of 8 months processed a working-memory (e.g., looking) task. Half of them were assessed again at age 4 with other working-memory tasks. The researchers concluded that in infants, cognitive processing is more widespread in the brain and processing becomes more localized at later ages, indicating brain specialization for cognitive processes. Infant emotional integration also has been a topic of research; researchers reported that 7-month-old infants reacted to two types of emotional information differently when they saw facial expressions of positive and negative emotions and heard emotionally congruent or incongruent vocal stimuli (Grossmann, Striano, & Friederici, 2006). Researchers concluded that infants of this age can recognize congruent and incongruent emotional affect across two modalities.

Review of Brain Development During the Toddler Years

One has only to observe a child of 12 to 30 months to understand the exponential growth of synaptic connections that occur during this age period. The brain growth spurt that began in infancy continues at a high pace throughout the toddler years and seems to correspond in time to the appearance of representational thinking, such as pretense and language (Epstein, 1978). By age 2, the number of synapses in the toddler brain reaches adult level, and by age 3 the brain has about 1,000 trillion synapses, which is twice the density of synapses present in the adult brain (Shore, 1997). The young brain also has a higher concentration of neurotransmitters, the communication facilitators of the brain, and the metabolic rate of the brain continues to increase. By age 2 the brain weighs about 3 pounds, and by age 3 the brain shows about 2.5 times as much activity as the adult brain. The increase in brain weight is partly due to the myelination by glial cells, which increases the speed of message transmission. Toddler-age children seem to be "biologically primed for learning" (Shore, 1997, p. 21; Meltzoff & Kuhl, 2016, p. 2). The toddler period is important for social, emotion, and language development as well as for cognitive development. For example, the emotional centers in the lower limbic system gain stronger connections with the frontal lobe of the brain, and this promotes toddlers' ability to understand and regulate emotions (Bergen & Woodin, 2011). The two major brain areas related to language development are active during this time period, with Broca's area having its greatest number of synapses and Wernike's area being almost completely myelinated by age 2 (Bergen & Woodin, 2011). Basic cognitive abilities such as attention and memory are well established by age 3, and young children show their increased cognitive understanding in early incongruous humor attempts (Bergen, 2015). According to Bornstein et al. (2006), the types and variations of experiences during the toddler years are related to later cognitive performance.

Research also indicates that the two hemispheres of the brain develop with slightly different patterns of activity. Chiron and colleagues' (1997) study of cerebral blood flow across the childhood age span, using the SPECT technique, noted that in 1-year-olds there appears to be a right hemisphere predominance. The amount of blood flow for the sensorimotor and parieto-temporal regions increases during the first three years, and these changes parallel behavior changes. For example, handedness is usually established between age 1 and 4 (related to brain hemispheric growth), sensory and motor control is established by age 3 to 4 (related to brain sensorimotor area growth), and perceptual and language growth spurts occur between ages 1 and 3 (related to development in the parieto-temporal areas involved in language). Memory development also is evident during the infant and toddler age period. There are many parts of the brain involved in memory; in fact, every neuron carries a memory! Although young infants have implicit memories stored in the lower and mid-brain area, explicit memories emerge more slowly since they depend on the maturation of the cerebral cortex (Eliot, 1999; Newcombe et al., 2014). New methods of research indicate that even infants are beginning to have longer-term memory (Bauer, 2002; Bauer et al., 2000). Usually in the early part of the second year, toddlers begin referring to explicit memories when they talk. This development is related to the primary areas in which memory is activated maturing and becoming myelinated. The hub of memory is in the medial temporal lobe, which houses the hippocampus, primarily responsible for long-term memory. Other developing areas involved in conscious memory are the medial thalamus and the basal forebrain, both of which store memories, and the prefrontal cortex, which is the site of source memory. By the age of 3, children can use their memory volitionally and learn memory strategies such as ordered repetition.

Studies of toddler brain development also show how various cognitive and other skills develop. For example, both *enactive* cognition (Bruner, 1964), involving understanding actions of real objects, and *iconic* cognition, involving pictures and symbols of objects, are developing during this age period. Researchers report that 18-month-old toddlers can differentiate familiar from unfamiliar objects when viewing them in both two and three dimensions, but those who saw real objects exhibited sensory differentiation more quickly than those who saw only pictures (Carver, Meltzoff, & Dawson, 2006). Carver and colleagues (2003) investigated the neural correlates of face recognition of familiar and unfamiliar faces and objects in children between 18 months and 54 months of age, and found that younger children showed a greater ERP response in the parietal area when looking at their mother's face while older children looked longer at the stranger's face. They concluded that the younger children were still developing parental attachment, but the older children had already established attachment so could focus more on other stimuli. In a review of brain areas involved in early language learning, particularly in the learning of more than one language, Kuhl (2010) outlined how infants' responses to phonetic stimuli are reflected in their later language and prereading abilities, and that this learning requires a "social context." She states, "Neuroscience on early language learning is beginning to reveal the multiple brain systems that underlie the human language faculty" (p. 713).

In discussing language and gesture imitation, Bates and Dick (2002, p. 12) stated that "the division of labor in the brain does not seem to break down neatly into language versus nonlanguage, nor is it neatly characterized by a split between comprehension (perception) versus production (action)." Bates and Dick (2002) conclude that initially there is no clear separation between the language and nonlanguage brain areas, and no clear split between perception and action. These authors report that there are significant positive correlations between the number of gestures young children correctly produce and independent measures of language production. For example, babbling is accompanied by rhythmic hand movements, naming by recognitory gestures, and word combinations by gesture-word and gesture-gesture combinations. The "vocabulary burst" that occurs at about 16–20 months is accompanied by a "comprehension burst" evidenced in both behavior measures and event-related brain potentials (ERP) (Goodman, 2001). By 30 months, when grammaticization is mastered, sequences of arbitrarily ordered gestures are evident (Bauer et al., 2000).

Impact of Genetic/Environmental Interactions During the First Three Years

Early achievements in brain development are determined by both genes and experience. Environmental enrichment may increase neuronal complexity, improve brain function, and facilitate recovery from brain injury, and these influences on specific abilities are more pronounced during critical or sensitive periods. Thus, environmental deprivation and/or stress during this early period may alter neuronal, hormonal, and immune systems and impair normal development, affecting children's physical, cognitive, and social-emotional abilities. Although, due to ethical reasons, experimental research is not possible, some "natural experiments" show correlations between stressful early environments and developmental delays; and children are more vulnerable to environmental deprivation, stress, or acquired insults during critical or sensitive periods (Perry, 1996). In a study of stress hormone regulation using cortisol samples taken from saliva, Carlson and Earls (1997) found that Romanian infants who were reared in institutions with the necessary food, shelter, and clothing but who lacked tactile and social interactions showed deficits in both physical growth and cognitive development at age 2. Developmental intervention conducted with a group of Romanian 2- and 3-year-olds showed that although intervention accelerated physical growth and mental/motor development in the intervention group compared to the control group, no cognitive differences were found. The cognitive scores for both groups were well below normal. In more recent studies, MRI scans of children who had been in severe institutional neglect conditions also showed there were brain size differences in certain areas, such as the amygdala (Mehta et al., 2009), and severe social-emotional neglect and/or abuse negatively affects brain development (Eluvathingal et al., 2006).

Maternal depression also may affect children's brain development. In a study of 11- to 17-month-old infants playing with their depressed and non-depressed mothers, Dawson and colleagues (1992) found that infants with depressed mothers had decreased left frontal EEG activity during the play and decreased right frontal activity during maternal separation. Other studies have shown behavior differences in such groups, such as less activity, shorter attention spans, and diminished motivation to master tasks (Dawson et al., 1994). Identification of structural and functional connections between the emotion and cognitive centers of the brain (e.g., between the amygdala and other parts of the limbic system and certain frontal lobe structures) suggests that there is a close connection between emotion and cognition, with emotional regulation centers of the brain serving as transmitters and monitors of cerebral functions related to thinking and learning. Greenspan (Greenspan & Lewis, 1999) has hypothesized that infants first learn to discriminate emotions and then learn cognitive categorization; that is, emotional development provides the basis for cognitive development. While this hypothesis needs further research, the early evidence suggests that there is a mediating influence of the limbic system (the site of basic emotions) on higher thought processing.

In a review of studies on effects of stress on brain development, Nelson and colleagues (1998, 2000) suggested that "plasticity in the developing brain represents a window of opportunity in normal circumstances, and represents a period of vulnerability in adverse circumstances" (1998, p. 79). Different factors present in "typical" family life may affect brain development. For example, researchers found that the types of words children spoke and their general vocabulary growth was related to the quantity of words spoken by their mothers (Huttenlocher, 1998; Tomasello, Mannie, & Kruger, 1996). Recent studies have indicated that mothers of varied socioeconomic classes may differ in the amount and complexity of speech to their children, and these differences have been associated with their children's speech richness or lack of richness (e.g. Hoff, 2003; Hoff & Tian, 2005). While such environmental differences may cause some developmental problems, there are other conditions that seem to have a high genetic component.

For example, one condition associated with issues in brain development in early life is that of autism spectrum disorder (ASD), which incorporates a range of severity levels in social skills, shows language delays, and may result in stereotyped repetitive behaviors. This disorder often has early manifestations and is usually diagnosed during the 2½- to 3-year age period, when a spurt of development in children's language and social skills should be evident. It may be initially suspected in young children's aversion to eye gaze (Pelphrey & McPartland, 2012) or to their lack of engagement in social or pretend play (Kasari et al., 2006). One hypothesis is that there may be a dysfunction in the amygdala centered system (Abell et al., 1999). That is, a disruption in the integrative functions of this system could account for emotional and social impairments and morphological abnormalities in the brain at later ages. Research has supported the finding that both the amygdala and the hippocampus may be enlarged in children with autistic symptoms (Sparks et al., 2002).

Other hypotheses address relationships between the cerebellum and the frontal lobe. Researchers (Harris et al., 1999) found that in children first diagnosed with autism at age 2 to 6, the ability to attend to stimuli was related to the size of the cerebellum (i.e., smaller cerebellum, poorer attention). Other studies have found a relationship between cerebellar motor functions and attention functions (Allen et al., 1997), and an inverse relationship between cerebellum size and frontal lobe size in children with autism (Carper & Courchesne, 2000). The developmental link between cerebellum and frontal lobe abnormalities may explain why impairments in higher-order thinking found in individuals with autism are persistent and pervasive. Courchesne and Pierce (2005) have suggested there may be over-connectivity in the frontal lobe and "connectivity between frontal cortex and other systems is poorly synchronized, weakly responsive, and information impoverished" (p. 225). Although much research is being conducted to understand this syndrome, there are still many unanswered questions.

There also has been research investigating the prevalence of autism spectrum characteristics in children diagnosed with Down syndrome. According to DiGuiseppi and colleagues (2010), autism spectrum disorder (ASD) is 17 to 20 times higher for children with Down than the estimated ASD prevalence in the general population. They indicate, however, that ASD also is associated with other disabilities. Down syndrome is a relatively common genetically-based syndrome, occurring in about 1 to 700–1,000 births. It is a chromosomal abnormality syndrome in which there is an extra chromosome (trisomy 21), and it results in some level of mental retardation. The syndrome involves impairments in many areas (e.g., cognitive, linguistic, social, emotional, motoric) and these impairments are evident even in the first few years of life. In an extensive review of characteristics of young children with this disability and suggested recommendations for treatment, Fidler (2005) has stressed that early intervention is important to enable them to develop optimally, especially building on their strengths in the areas of visual processing, receptive language, and social skills. She advises educators to promote development of their "visual processing and visual-motor coordination, as well as their relative strengths in social functioning and forming social relationships" and suggests that "promotion of strengths in targeted ways may facilitate the bootstrapping of weaker skills" (p. 98).

Suggestions for Fostering Brain Development and Learning in the Early Years

Because synaptic growth is intense during this age period, enriched environmental features should be available. Toddlers are ready to "go out and meet the world" and enjoy new experiences. However, their judgment regarding safety and caution is not well developed, so the environment must ensure both challenge and safety.

For Families

- Family environments with basic health and care requirements (food, shelter, and other essentials) should be available for all young children. Families should seek services if they lack resources to provide them.
- Because these years are so important for children's brain development, families should provide emotionally safe and cognitively stimulating experiences for their young children in the home and through cultural opportunities in the community.
- If care outside the family is needed, family members should seek care environments that provide not only basic health and social-emotional safety, but also cognitive stimulation to foster their children's optimum brain development.

For Educarers and Educators

- Because young children's development co-occurs with significant changes in brain structure and function, educarers can encourage young children's active manipulation of objects, scaffold their mastery of developmental milestones, and provide opportunities for varied experiences. Each child's progress should be monitored regularly, and feedback to parents about child growth should be provided.
- High-quality child care and education programs (e.g., high adult-to-child ratios, small class size, nurturing environments, play-oriented experiences) should be provided. Quality programs are especially important for young children from high-risk family environments.
- Children with early identified disabilities (e.g., Down syndrome, autism spectrum disorder) especially benefit from educare activities that enhance the growth of the brain. Because claims for specific types of environments for certain developmental problems are not supported by research evidence, professionals' involvement in research studies that test environmental effects is encouraged.

For Community Partners and Policy Makers

- Families who need assistance in providing excellent care and educational experiences for their young children should be identified, and public policies that enable them to get that assistance should be established.

- Standards such as child-staff ratios, appropriate equipment, and staff training for infant and toddler educarers should be clearly stated and enforced by governmental units at all levels.
- Children who need special assistance because of disabilities that may influence brain and other areas of development should be a special focus of public concern. To meet the needs of these children, their families should have financial and other types of support.

Case 3 Tasha's Toddler Development (Down's)

Because Tasha's mother became pregnant at age 45, Tasha's parents decided to have a prenatal amniocentesis examination, and they were told that she had Down's syndrome (trisomy 21, which is an extra chromosome). They learned as much as they could about this condition and contacted community resources early, so they have had good assistance in understanding and supporting Tasha's development. She is now a stocky 2-year-old who has a sunny disposition, and her mother states that she was an "easy" baby, having regular eating and sleeping habits. She responded well during infant/parent play by cooing and babbling, seemed to understand both motor and verbal cues, and vocalized when playing with objects. However, she began to show motor, language, and cognitive delays by the latter part of her first year. She did not roll over purposefully until 9 months, did not sit alone until 12 months, and did not crawl until 15 months. At 18 months, she has only recently begun walking around the furniture and standing briefly alone. Her fine motor skills have developed well and her social skills are a strong point. However, she has only a few spoken words at this point and her articulation is poor. Her cognitive skills also seem to be more like those of a 1-year-old. She enjoys play with parents and siblings, is outgoing and friendly to visitors, and has benefitted from time in an early intervention program that has both children who are typically developing and those who have special needs. Tasha has been involved in early intervention since birth, receiving physical and occupational therapy as well as speech therapy. Her parents are pleased with her progress and with the assistance they have received from the various service providers. However, they are concerned about Tasha's long-term development, especially her cognitive development, and they want her to be treated first as an individual and not as a "Down's child." They want Tasha to have opportunities to learn as much as she can and don't want low expectations for her development. She is scheduled for participation in a form of child evaluation called Transdisciplinary Play-Based Assessment (Linder & Linas, 2009).

Case 4 Liam's Toddler Development (Incipient Autism)

When Asha's aunt, Dena, first visited her niece and her husband, Marco, and met their 5- month-old baby, Liam, she became a little concerned because Liam did not try to gain eye contact with her. He averted his gaze whenever she tried to gain eye contact, and Dena's own children had always looked directly at her when she interacted with them. Since neither of Liam's parents seemed to notice this lack of eye gaze, however, Dena did not mention her concern to them. Because she lived far away, she was not able to see Liam on a regular basis and his parents did not mention any problems they were having during his early development. However, when Liam was 11 months old, both Asha and Marco began to have some concerns about Liam's interactions with objects in play because they were very repetitive and extended. Also, he did not seem responsive to their social and language interactions or exhibit positive emotions or enjoyment. Liam's play often focused on spinning various toys or doing other repetitive types of actions, and he did not respond to their attempts to enlarge his play behaviors. These behaviors seemed even more problematic a few months later when Liam was 15 months old, because when Asha tried to have him engage in pretend actions, he did not seem to understand pretense but remained literal in his interactions with both people and objects. His language also was not developing well, and he did not show many attempts to communicate with other children. He did show extended interest in using Marco's electronic tablet though, and would spend as much time on the tablet as he was allowed. Aunt Dena visited that year at the time of Liam's 2-year-old birthday, and in response to some concerns that Asha expressed, Dena then ventured a suggestion that Liam might be showing behaviors that are common in children on the autism spectrum. She suggested that his parents should have an evaluation made since there were ways to help him if he did have autistic tendencies. His parents were surprised and very upset by Dena's comment, however, so she is not sure whether they will follow through on her suggestion.

Study Guide/Questions for Discussion

- Review the information on brain development in the toddler years and identify five important ways that development of various parts of the brain is demonstrated in toddlers' expanding repertoire of behaviors.
- Compare the development of Dana, Cody, Tasha, and Liam. List what they have in common and what is different about their development, and suggest steps their parents can take to promote their healthy development. Indicate resources that could help them.
- Using information on toddler development, explain how parents and teachers can provide environments that support and encourage the development of language, cognitive, and social skills in toddlers.
- Discuss how various child care arrangements (at home, with another family, in daycare) can all provide good environments for healthy brain development during the toddler years.
- Identify societal implications of having toddlers with special needs provided with services they need to assist their optimum development.

Bibliography

Abell, F., Krama, M., Ashburner, J., Passingham, R., Firston, K., Frackowiak, R., Happe, F., Frith, C., & Grith, U. (1999). The neuroanatomy of autism: A voxel-based whole brain analysis of structural scans. *Neuroreport, 10*(8), 1647–1651.

Allen, G., Buxton, R. B., Wong, E. C., & Courchesne, E. (1997). Attentional activation of the cerebellum independent of motor involvement. *Science, 275*, 1940–1943.

Bates, E., & Dick, F. (2002). Language, gesture, and the developing brain. *Developmental Psychobiology, 40*(3), 293–310.

Bauer, P. J. (2002). Long—term recall memory: Behavioral and neuro—developmental changes in the first 2 years of life. *Current Directions in Psychological Science, 11*(4), 137–141.

Bauer, P. J., Wenner, J. A., Dropik, P. L., & Wewerka, S. S. (2000). Parameters of remembering and forgetting in the transition from infamy to early childhood. *Monographs of the Society for Research in Child Development, 65*(4), Serial # 263.

Bell, A., & Wolfe, C. (2007). Changes in brain function from infancy to early childhood: Evidence from EEG power and coherence during working memory tasks. *Developmental Neuropsychology, 31*(1), 21–38.

Bergen, D. (2015). Play as a context for humor development. In D. Fromberg & D. Bergen (Eds.), *Play from birth to twelve: Contexts, perspectives, and meaning* (3rd ed., pp. 159–172). New York: Routledge.

Bergen, D., & Woodin, M. (2011). Neuropsychological development of newborns, infants, and toddlers. In A. S. Davis (Ed.), *Handbook of pediatric neuropsychology* (pp. 15–30). New York: Springer.

Bornstein, M. H., Hahn, C., Bell, C., Haynes, O. M., Slater, A., Golding, J., . . . ALSPAC Study Team. (2006). Stability in cognition across early childhood: A developmental cascade. *Psychological Science, 17*(2), 151–158.

Bruner, J. S. (1964). The course of cognitive growth. *American Psychologist, 19*(1), 1–15. doi:10.1037/h0044160.

Carlson, M., & Earls, F. (1997). Psychological and neuroendocrinological sequelae of early social deprivation in institutionalized children in Romania. In C. S. Carter, I. I. Lederhendler, & B. Kirkpatrick (Eds.), *The integrative neurobiology of affiliation* (pp. 419–428). New York: New York Academy of Sciences.

Carper, R. A., & Courchesne, E. (2000). Inverse correlation between frontal lobe and cerebellum sizes in children with autism. *Brain, 123*(4), 836–844.

Carver, L. J., Dawson, G., Panagiotides, H., Meltzoff, A. N., McPartland, J., Gray, J., & Munson, J. (2003). Age-related differences in neural correlates of face recognition during the toddler and preschool years. *Developmental Psychology, 42*, 143–159.

Carver, L. J., Meltzoff, A. N., & Dawson, G. (2006). Event-related potential (ERP) indices of infants' recognition of familiar and unfamiliar objects in two and three dimensions. *Developmental Science, 9*(1), 51–62.

Chiron, C., Jambaque, I., Nabbout, R., Lounes, R., Syrota, A., & Dulac, O. (1997). The right brain hemisphere is dominant in human infants. *Brain, 120*(6), 1057–1065.

Coude, G., Festante, F., Cilla, A., Lolacono, V., Bimbi, M., Fogassi, L., & Francesco Ferrari, P. (2016). Mirror neurons of ventral premotor cortex are modulated by social cues provided by others' gaze. *The Journal of Neuroscience, 36*(11), 3145–3156.

Courchesne, E., & Pierce, K. (2005). Why the frontal cortex in autism might be talking only to itself: Local over-connectivity but long-distance disconnection. *Current Opinion in Neurobiology, 15*(2), 225–230.

Dawson, G., Hessl, D., & Frey, K. (1994). Social influences on early developing biological and behavioral systems related to risk for affective disorder. *Development and Psychopathology, 6*(4), 759–779.

Dawson, G., Klinger, L., Panagiotides, H., Hill, D., & Spieker, S. (1992). Frontal lobe activity and affective behavior of infants of mothers with depressive symptoms. *Child Development, 63*, 725–737.

Dawson, G., Meltzoff, A. N., Osterling, J., & Rinaldi, J. (1998). Neuropsychological correlates of early symptoms of autism. *Child Development, 69*(5), 1276–1285.

DiGuiseppi, C., Hepburn, S., Davis, J. M., Fidler, D. J., Hartway, S., Lee, N. R., . . . Robinson, C. (2010). Screening for autism spectrum disorders in children with Down syndrome: Population prevalence and screening test characteristics. *Journal of Developmental and Behavioral Pediatrics: JDBP, 31*(3), 181.

Eliot, L. (1999). *What's going on in there? How the brain and mind develop in the first five-years of life*. New York: Bantam.

Elsabbagh, M., Mercure, E., Hudry, K., Chandler, S., Pasco, G., Charman, T., . . . BASIS Team. (2012). Infant neural sensitivity to dynamic eye gaze is associated with later emerging autism. *Current Biology, 22*(4), 338–342.

Eluvathingal, T. J., Chugani, H. T., Behen, M. E., Juhász, C., Muzik, O., Maqbool, M., . . . Makki, M. (2006). Abnormal brain connectivity in children after early severe socioemotional deprivation: A diffusion tensor imaging study. *Pediatrics, 117*(6), 2093–2100.

Epstein, H. (1978). Growth spurts during brain development: Implications for educational policy and practice. In J. Chall & A. Mirsky (Eds.), *Education and the brain, 77th National Society for the study of education yearbook*. Chicago: Chicago University Press.

Fidler, D. J. (2005). The emerging Down syndrome behavioral phenotype in early childhood: Implications for practice. *Infants & Young Children, 18*(2), 86–103.

Percaccio, C. R., Conboy, B. T., Romo, H., Klarman, L., Ortiz, S., & Kuhl. P. K., (2011). Bilingual language learning: An ERP study relating early brain responses to speech, language input, and later word production. *Journal of Phonetics, 39*(4), 546–557.

Goodman, J. C. (2001, April). The rate and shape of receptive and expressive vocabulary development in infants and toddlers. Paper presented at the *Society for Research in Child Development*, Minneapolis, MN.

Greenspan, S. I., & Lewis, N. B. (1999). *Building healthy minds: The six experiences that create intelligence and emotional growth in babies and young children*. Cambridge, MA: Perseus.

Grossmann, T., Striano, T., & Friederici, A. D. (2006). Crossmodal integration of emotional information from face and voice in the infant brain. *Developmental Science, 9*(3), 309–315.

Harris, N. S., Courchesne, E., Townsend, J., Carper, R. A., & Lord, C. (1999). Neuroanatomic contributions to slowed orienting of attention in children with autism. *Cognitive Brain Research, 8*(1), 61–71.

Hoff, E. (2003). The specificity of environmental influence: Socioeconomic status affects early vocabulary development via maternal speech. *Child Development, 74*(5), 1368–1378.

Hoff, E., & Tian, C. (2005). Socioeconomic status and cultural influences on language. *Journal of Communication Disorders, 38*(4), 271–278.

Huttenlocher, J. (1998). Language input and language growth. *Preventive Medicine: An International Journal Devoted to Practice & Theory, 27*(2), 195–199.

Kasari, C., Freeman, S., & Paparella, T. (2006). Joint attention and symbolic play in young children with autism: A randomized controlled intervention study. *Journal of Child Psychology and Psychiatry, 47*(6), 611–620.

Kiester, E. (2001). Accents are forever. *Smithsonian, 31*(10), 14–15.

Kuhl, P. K. (2010). Brain mechanisms in early language acquisition. *Neuron, 67*(5), 713–727.

Linder, T., & Linas, K. (2009). A functional, holistic approach to developmental assessment through play: The transdisciplinary play-based assessment. *Zero to Three (J), 30*(1), 28–33.

Mehta, M. A., Golembo, N. I., Nosarti, C., Colvert, E., Mota, A., Williams, S. C., . . . Sonuga-Barke, E. J. (2009). Amygdala, hippocampal and corpus callosum size following severe early institutional deprivation: The English and Romanian Adoptees study pilot. *Journal of Child Psychology and Psychiatry, 50*(8), 943–951.

Meltzoff, A. N., & Kuhl, P. K. (2016). Exploring the infant social brain: What's going on in there? *Connecting Science, Policy, and Practice*, 2–9.

Nelson, C. A., & Carver, L. J. (1998). The effects of stress and trauma on brain and memory: A view from developmental cognitive neuroscience. *Development and Psychopathology, 10*(4), 793–809.

Nelson, C. A., Monk, C. S., Lin, J., Carver, L. J., Thomas, K. M., & Truwit, C. L. (2000). Functional neuroanatomy of spatial working memory in children. *Developmental Psychology, 36*(1), 109–116.

Newcombe, N. S., Balcomb, F., Ferrara, K., Hansen, M., & Koski, J. (2014). Two rooms, two representations? Episodic-like memory in toddlers and preschoolers. *Developmental Science, 17*, 743–756.

Pelphrey, K. A., & McPartland, J. C. (2012). Brain development: Neural signatures predicts autism's emergence. *Current Biology, 22*, 3–4. doi:10.10.161j.cub.2012.01.025.

Perry, B. D. (1996). Incubated in terror: Neurodevelopmental factors in the 'cycle of violence.' In J. D. Osofsky (Ed.), *Children, youth and violence: Searching for solutions* (pp. 2–20). New York: Guilford.

Rizzolatti, G., & Craighero, L. (2004). The mirror-neuron system. *Annual Review of Neuroscience, 27*, 169–192.

Shore, R. (1997). *Rethinking the brain: New insights into early development*. New York: Families and Work Institute.

Sparks, B. F., Friedman, S. D., Shaw, D. W., Aylward, E. H., Echelard, D., Artru, A. A., . . . Dager, S. R. (2002). Brain structural abnormalities in young children with autism spectrum disorder. *Neurology, 59*(2), 184–192.

Thompson, R. A., & Nelson, C. A. (2001). Developmental science and the media: Early brain development. *American Psychologist, 56*(1), 5–15.

Tomasello, M., Mannie, S., & Kruger, A. C. (1996). Linguistic environment of 1- to 2-year-old twins. *Developmental Psychology, 22*(20), 169–176.

Weber, C., Hahne, A., Friedrich, M., & Friederici, A. D. (2004). Discrimination of word stress in early infant perception: Electrophysiological evidence. *Cognitive Brain Research, 18*(2), 149–161.

Weismer, S. E., Lord, C., & Esler, A. (2010). Early language patterns of toddlers on the autism spectrum compared to toddlers with developmental delay. *Journal of Autism and Developmental Disorders, 40*(10), 1259–1273.

5

BRAIN DEVELOPMENT AND LEARNING IN THE PRESCHOOL YEARS

Case 1 Lonnie's Autonomy Development

Lonnie's parents have enjoyed every minute of his life until very recently. His birth was without complications, he nursed well, accepted other food when it was offered, and went through the typical developmental milestones during his early years. His personality was adaptable, engaging, and emotionally mild, and he took to new experiences very easily. His parents were fortunate because both of their sets of parents could care for him, so his mother was able to go back to work early. Lonnie started preschool the same week as his third birthday, and at first he seemed to adapt very well. His teachers remarked on his engaging personality, initiative, and adaptability to the new experiences, and he gained some "buddies" easily in the preschool classroom. He had a great imagination, enjoyed pretending to be media characters, and loved playing with trucks and blocks. Right about the time of his fourth birthday, his parents and grandparents noted a change in behavior that concerned them. Lonnie began refusing the food he had always eaten, insisting on having his favorite blue cup and resisting drinking from a cup of another color, and saying "no" to many directions that the adults gave him. When his parents mentioned these changed behaviors to the teachers, they indicated that they also had noted some of this behavior at preschool. However, they explained that children of 4 or 4 ½ often become less compliant to adult demands and want to try out their own "power." They suggested that the adults give him more opportunities for choosing his actions (within limits) as the teachers do with the 4-year-olds in their classroom.

Case 2 Joe's Attention Problems

Joe also started out developing well, and in his first few years his development was not of concern to his parents, although he was always a very active child. He crawled and walked at 9 months, had many short-term interests, and showed affection easily. When he turned 3, his mother was busy with a new baby and so she often let Joe entertain himself in their yard. He spent a great deal of time outside riding his tricycle on the driveway, jumping on a little trampoline, climbing on the steps, kicking a ball around the yard, or chasing the dog around the yard. When Joe's dad was home, he and his son engaged in "roughhouse" types of play that Joe really seemed to enjoy. Joe's mother noticed that when he had to stay inside and needed to entertain himself, he did not spend very much time on any activity. In fact, his iPad was the only toy that he would play with for more than a few minutes. When he started preschool at age 4, his teacher said that his behavior was very active and often unfocused. Joe's typical behavior is moving quickly around the room and interacting with various toys and materials very briefly. At group time, he has difficulty sitting and attending to the activity for more than 5 minutes and he does not stay seated at the table during snack time. His teacher is wondering if Joe might have an attention deficit because of his inability to concentrate on teacher-directed and sometimes even on self-chosen activities. While this type of behavior is not unusual in 4-year-olds, since Joe will be 5 in another month, the teacher had expected his attention span to expand in length as it has for most of the 4-year-olds in the class. The teacher expected that by age 5, he would be able to control his attention, focus on what the teacher says in group activities, and stay with tasks that require persistence and care. Joe's teacher has suggested to the family that Joe should be evaluated for this "attention-deficit" condition as he may need medication to help him be able to pay attention in kindergarten.

Review of Brain Development During the Preschool Years

This period continues the phase of rapid growth of the brain and thus also continues the period of major environmental vulnerability, especially in relation to development of language and intellectual systems. There is some preliminary but controversial evidence that neurons may continue to be generated, with cortical neurons possibly doubling between age 15 months and 6 years (Shankle et al., 1998). From ages 3 to 6, synaptogenesis (development of new synapses) continues rapidly, and by age 4 cerebral metabolic rates of glucose utilization are two times normal adult levels (Chugani et al., 2008). Cerebral size levels off during this age period (Giedd et al., 1996). Myelination also continues in some brain areas during the 3 to 6 age period, for example, in portions of the limbic system. Chiron et al. (1997) found that during age 3 to 5, there are also change points in cerebral blood flow levels, with a change beginning at age 5 for hemispheres, at age 3 for sensorimotor areas, and at age 3 for parieto-temporal regions, signaling further refinements in fine motor, sensory-gross motor, memory, and language skills. Source memory, which is awareness of where and when something was learned, emerges in the latter part of this age period, coinciding with maturation of the frontal lobe (Eliot, 1999). Thompson and colleagues (Thompson et al., 2001) scanned brain growth patterns of children age 3 to 15 over four years and reported that the 3 to 6 age period shows the fastest growth rates in the frontal networks that regulate planning of new actions. As noted earlier, young children's language development processes are related to specific areas of brain development, and this is especially apparent during the preschool years. Ortiz-Mantilla et al. (2010) found significant and consistent correlations between amygdala size and language abilities. They report that typically developing 6-month-old infants with larger right amygdalae have consistently lower receptive and expressive language scores at age 2, 3, and 4, and they state, "the amygdala might play an important but as yet unspecified role in mediating language acquisition" (p. 2791). However, children with injuries involving the left temporal lobes have delays in both vocabulary and grammar production, and use more gestures as a compensatory behavior. Bates and Dick (2002) state,

> Perception and production of gesture and language travel at the same time (over development) and in the same places (in the brain). However, these fellow travelers sometimes stage a dramatic breakup, as seen in studies of normal children, late talkers, and children with focal brain injury.
>
> *(p. 9)*

These theorists indicate that sensorimotor organization, stages of observation and perception, age and expertise, and the amount of context provided will all affect young children's language development. According to Fletcher (2011), preschool children's social development, language growth, and increases in symbolic representation can be observed in their interactions with peers and in their advanced levels of pretend play. She suggests that play settings provide a setting in which emotional regulation, control of aggression, and exhibition of pro-social behaviors can be developed.

In studies using ERP technology, Tan and Molfese (2009), who looked at how preschool-age children discriminated between words of different syntactic classes, found that when the children looked at videos in which the language matched or failed to match the actions and objects of a person doing various actions with toys, the preschoolers showed wavelengths at some P100 and N220 sites that discriminated among the different syntactic classes for both match and mismatch situations. They did not have the same capability as adults, however. In a study of attention processes and executive functioning skills at this age level, Liu et al. (2009) found evidence for activity in the prefrontal cortex associated with the development of reasoning ability. They studied 4- to 6-year-old children's brain waves as they reasoned about reality and false-belief questions in animated videos and found a difference in the LSW (left scalp) distribution between children who failed and passed false-belief questions. Children with false-belief knowledge reasoned similarly to adults about the characters' beliefs.

A few studies have generated hypotheses about the relationship of brain activity to temperament and behavior in the 3 to 5 age period. For example, frontal lobe activity during preschoolers' play has been studied by Fox and colleagues (1995, 1996) and their findings indicate that highly social children with right frontal EEG asymmetry were more likely to have externalizing problems than highly social children with left frontal EEG asymmetry. Further, shy children with increased right frontal EEG asymmetry showed more internalizing problems than did those with left frontal EEG asymmetry. Fox and colleagues proposed that many cognitive processes may be mediated by areas within the frontal lobe and that children with greater left frontal asymmetry may be better prepared to regulate affective arousal. No conclusions can be reached without confirming studies, however.

Some studies have compared the brain development effects of preschoolers' training on various tasks. Rueda, Rothbart and colleagues (2005) investigated the efficiency of attentional networks after training by comparing trained and untrained 4- and 6-year-olds; they found that training and age were relevant, and that both the anterior cingulate and lateral prefrontal areas were involved in this process. Also, in music training for Head Start children, Neville and colleagues (2008) found that the children who received music training were better at showing auditory selective attention (increase in ERPs in response to the stimuli).

In a recent review by Brown and Jernigan (2012) of preschool children's brain development, they note that both structural growth and morphological changes are extensive, with increases in the cortical area, changing cortical volume, gray and white matter tissue changes, and increasing metabolic demands. They confirm that a greater number of brain regions are required for young children to complete cognitive tasks, and they note that this "scaffolding" is eliminated with increasing age. They urge more study of this age level because there are fewer studies compared to the number of studies of infant brain development, and they conclude that

> The preschool years can be thought of as a developmental period generally dominated by dynamic and robust progressive processes, with an emphasis on growth, expansion, "construction," and "blossoming" that will later be pruned and tuned with continued maturation and experience.
>
> *(Brown & Jernigan, 2012, p. 18)*

Impact of Genetic/Environmental Interactions During the Preschool Years

Although there is expansive and positive evidence about the dynamics of brain development during the preschool years, it also is clear that the impact of poor environmental conditions, especially abusive conditions, can have particularly deleterious effects on children of this age level (and other age levels). Brain differences resulting from abuse and neglect during this age period may have long-lasting physical, cognitive, motivational, and social-emotional effects. In a recent review of effects of childhood abuse of all types, Anda and colleagues (2006) indicate that most of the nation's efforts to remediate societal health and behavioral problems must be viewed within their "common origins in the enduring neurodevelopmental consequences of abuse and related adverse experiences during childhood" (p. 11). For example, there is evidence that abused children often show a different pattern of electrical activity in the frontal and temporal lobes (in the site of limbic system functions). Also, children exposed to the severe stress of abuse have exhibited strong physiological responses, even to minimal stress conditions at later ages (Perry, 1996). According to Perry, extreme trauma may affect brain-stem areas that regulate immediate responses related to biological survival, making them "overdevelop" while restricting the development of cortical and limbic areas, which control higher-order thinking and emotions. Thus, it is possible that the impulsivity, hyperactivity, and poor affect regulation often seen in children from abusive environments is evidence of a distortion in brain development. Also, the hippocampus may be atrophied in children who endure abusive situations, resulting in long-term memory deficits (Bremner et al., 1997). In a study of children who had been sexually abused in early childhood (DeBellis et al., 1999), the researchers found that at school age, these children had smaller brain volume and larger lateral ventricles, and there was less development of the corpus callosum. Moreover, the length of the abuse correlated with the extensiveness of the brain structural differences. Hart and Rubia (2012), in a review of neuroimaging studies of child abuse, indicate that deficits in IQ, memory, working memory, attention, response inhibition, and emotion discrimination are all associated with evidence of abuse. These studies show that brain volume, gray and white matter distribution in the dorsolateral and ventromedial prefrontal cortex, hippocampus, amygdala, and corpus callosum show deficits, and diffusion tensor imaging (DTI) studies indicate neural network deficiencies. In another review of brain development effects of abuse, McCrory, DeBrito, and Viding (2012) note that, while evidence of harm to various brain areas is not always consistent, both ERP and fMRI studies have noted that maltreated children often are hypervigilant regarding potential social threats, which may "be at the cost of other developmental processes" (p. 154). Eliot (1999) has stated that it is in the brain where "the real scars of child abuse and neglect lie" (p. 325). She notes that concerns about effects on brain development from abusive environmental conditions are particularly of concern for children age birth to 6, because as a brain region passes its pruning stage,

> The opportunity to rewire it is significantly limited. The critical periods for basic sensory abilities, like vison and hearing, end much earlier than those for more complex skills, like language and emotion, whose underlying neural circuits prune their synapses and myelinate their axons over most of childhood. [Nevertheless] all critical periods probably begin within the first four years of life, when the synaptic tide turns from waxing to waning in all brain areas.
>
> *(p. 38)*

Research has indicated that child maltreatment and early trauma experiences also may be linked to other brain conditions, such as attention deficit hyperactivity disorder (ADHD) and oppositional defiant behavior (ODD) (see Ford et al., 2000). The pattern of neuropsychological behavior in ADHD children seems to be related to executive functions and working memory, which are sited in the frontal lobe, and some neuroimaging studies have implicated fronto-subcortical pathways, which are rich in catecholamines, components of the drugs used in treating ADHD (Faraone & Biederman, 1998). Potential neurological development differences in young children with ADHD have been studied extensively in young children, and recent studies indicate that both white and gray matter areas are affected (Castellanos et al., 2002), resulting in executive disfunction and delay aversion differences compared to controls (Sonuga-Barke et al., 2003). In longitudinal studies, however, growth curves of these children are similar to controls, with the exception of the caudate nucleus, and thus their brain growth seems typical in later childhood and adolescence (Castellanos et al., 2002). Panksepp (1998) has discussed this less mature development of the frontal lobes of children with ADHD and theorized that since this lobe is primarily responsible for inhibition of action, planning, and conceptualization of complex tasks, a longer period of active rough and tumble play, which these young children seem to need, may be facilitative of their frontal lobe development. He suggests that children with ADHD may need longer periods and more extensive levels of such play; that is, that their behavior is signaling that they need more time for active play. He speculates that, when ADHD children are given drugs that inhibit activity and make them passive, this treatment may be inhibiting their frontal lobe development. Given the number of young children being diagnosed and treated with drugs, this hypothesis needs further research, especially since playground researchers are finding children now have fewer opportunities for active recess play at school (Pellegrini & Bjorklund, 1996).

Preschool experiences as ameliorators of environmental deficiencies have been advocated for over 30 years, since the initiation of Head Start, and there have been many studies reporting some areas of long-term effectiveness (see Zigler & Bishop-Josef, 2006). Many longitudinal research studies on the effects of high-quality child care and preschool experiences for low-income children have indicated that there were long-term positive effects in social skills, attention, and task performance (see Belsky et al., 2007; Hill, Gormley, & Adelstein, 2012; Peisner-Feinberg et al., 2001; Reynolds, Magnuson, & Ou, 2010; Schweinhart, 1993; Nores et al., 2005). Findings show that fewer children who participate in such programs are identified as having special needs, and more perform successfully in school and graduate from high school. Also, fewer are incarcerated. The benefits seem to be primarily directed to self-regulation, attention, language, and other school-related skills that support higher academic performance, although an actual increase in intelligence has not been reported (see te Nijenhuis, Jongeneel-Grimen, & Kirkegaard, 2014). Presently, extensive research on the brain development of young children who are preschool program participants has not been conducted, so it is unclear how brain synaptic connections or other changes in brain structure and function may be promoted by these programs. It may be that the major function of such programs is to increase the amount of time that young children from low-income, abusive, or unchallenging environments are able to spend in more supportive and appropriately challenging environments.

Suggestions for Fostering Brain Development and Learning in Years 3 to 5

For Families

- Because development of a dense neuronally connected and integrated brain occurs at this age, families should provide environmental support and experiences to enhance that development. This includes good nutrition, safe exploration areas, warm and supportive encouragement, and diverse enjoyable and challenging experiences for their children.
- Families should talk to children extensively using a varied and elaborated vocabulary and be responsive to their children's language attempts. This will

promote children's school learning experiences because they will begin with a strong language and knowledge base. Since preschools also support young children's learning and development, families should investigate quality and choose ones that meet early childhood standards.

- Parents can help their children learn the alphabet, numbers, and basic colors, not by "direct teaching" but by reading to their children often and seeking everyday activities (e.g., in grocery stores, while driving, at sporting activities) to talk about experiences, point out and read signs, and engage in numeracy activities such as counting and estimating objects.
- Because environments of abuse and/or neglect are harmful to children at any age, but especially at this age, families should avoid such behaviors. If one partner in the family shows these types of behavior, the other partner should seek help to protect the children. If neglect is due to financial problems, families should obtain needed nutritional and other supports from relevant agencies.

For Educators

- Educators working with these children should provide environments with many opportunities for social-emotional, physical-sensory-motor, and language-cognition experiences to promote the development of new synaptic connections. They should encourage mastery experiences both in play as well as in "real-world" tasks. Young children need many opportunities to use emerging skills to strengthen their existing synaptic connections in areas important for educational success (e.g., language, memory).
- Because most early childhood educators now work in inclusive environments, they need to stay informed about brain research and suggestions for working with children with disabilities as well as for typically developing children. Active learning environments that assist typically developing children can also expand the development of children with special needs. Early childhood educators and early childhood special educators should work as partners during the preschool years.
- Children diagnosed with ADHD can be given natural supports for gaining control over their activity levels, and these supports, rather than drugs, are preferable whenever possible. Because there are questions about long-term effects of drugs that inhibit motor behavior on brain growth and neurological development, allowing these children to have active play and higher levels of motor activity is a better way to further the development of their motor and frontal lobe functions.

For Community Partners and Policy Makers

- Community partners should be aware of the early education opportunities their communities provide and promote local, state, federal, and private sources of funding to ensure all young children have optimal opportunities for excellent brain development.

- Advocacy for positive, emotionally safe environments and high-quality experiences for all children are warranted, given the fact that negative effects of extremely poor environments are already documented by brain research.
- Support for adequate funding levels for preschool programs and for high standards of training for preschool teachers is warranted. Also, advocacy for higher salary levels for such teachers should be strong.
- Public policy that supports families that are in stressful situations is warranted, since family stress can result in abusive or otherwise stressful environments for young children and this can have long-term consequences.

Case 3 Marie's Language Problems

At age 3 ½, Maria is a placid and agreeable child who follows directions well and engages for long times in self-chosen activities. She seemed to develop normally during her first year and her physical and cognitive development was typical at that time. Her parents have indicated that they used sign language during her earlier years because she did not begin to say any words even when she was age 1 ½, and they reported her understanding of and use of the sign language was excellent. She now is beginning to use spoken language, but she speaks familiar words with poor enunciation. Her one- and two-word sentences are difficult to understand, and she has not yet begun to talk in well-formed sentences. At age 2, her parents became concerned because of this lack of progress in speaking, so they had her hearing evaluated and found that her auditory capabilities were in the normal range. Because the range of normality for language production is wide, they were advised to "give her more time." However, when she turned age 3, an evaluation by a speech therapist showed her expressive language was in the 18- to 20-month category. She still has a small range of sentences that she uses often and her enunciation continues to be poor. The therapist indicated that she had difficulty using the back of her tongue to form words. Marie is not disinterested in speaking, however, as she is socially engaged with others and makes speaking attempts that are often not understood. Her interest in communicating but lack of success in doing so has resulted recently in a tendency for tantrums. Her parents are concerned that their usually happy child will change if her language difficulties are not soon addressed. Therefore, based on the speech therapist's evaluation, her parents have decided to enroll her in intensive speech therapy.

Case 4 Bucky's Experiences and an Educator's Dilemma

At the child care program where Ms. Darden worked, there are children from a wide variety of families. Many of them are single parents who work two or three different jobs in order to keep their families together. Lina Waley is one such parent, and when she enrolled her son Bucky into the program, she said he would be there usually from 8 a.m. to 4 p.m. for five days a week—but there were many days when he did not arrive. There always seemed to be emergencies or injuries in which Bucky was involved, and sometimes he came to child care wearing bandages. Bucky's behavior on those days was problematic also. Sometimes he lashed out at other children or isolated himself and refused to participate in activities. One day when Bucky was wearing long pants and a long-sleeved shirt, he complained about being too hot, and so Ms. Darden helped him roll up his pants and shirt sleeves. That was when she noticed that Bucky's arms and one leg were covered with bruises. She asked Bucky what had happened, but he ignored her question and said "I want to go play," so she did not pursue any more questions. However, she did discuss the incident with the owner of the center, and they decided that they needed to document what they were seeing and perhaps report their concerns to Children's Services. Later that week when Lina arrived to pick up Bucky, Ms. Darden again asked about Bucky's injuries and Lina became angry and said, "He just falls a lot and fights a lot. He is a really bad kid" and she whisked him quickly away. A few days later when it was time for Bucky to leave the center, his mother did not arrive. An hour later, Lina's mother came to pick up Bucky and she said that Lina had been in a fight with her boyfriend and so was not feeling well enough to pick up Bucky. Ms. Darden and her supervisor are now trying to decide what their next step should be since they are not sure whether this "boyfriend" is the one who harmed Bucky. They think that his home environment is not a good one for him, but they don't really want to be in a battle with this family. On the other hand, they have a responsibility to report child abuse if that is happening to Bucky.

Study Guide/Questions for Discussion

- The 3 to 5 age period is a major time of synaptogenesis, especially in the frontal lobes of the brain. State how this growth might be reflected in children's social, emotional, and cognitive development.
- What might be happening in Lonnie's brain at the age of 4 that could be reflected in his new behaviors of autonomy and resistance to adult direction? Would this be considered typical behavior at this age? Why or why not?
- Should Joe's parents be concerned about his short attention span, or is that not unusual for a child of this age? Identify three "ordinary" activities to help children with attention problems to use natural supports and gain better control over their activity levels and suggest one of these that might help Joe.
- Discuss when Maria's parents should have her language abilities evaluated. Do they also need her hearing evaluated? When would speech therapy be appropriate for her, given the wide range of normality in age for speech development?
- List some interventions to reduce child abuse for children such as Bucky. Plan a talk about what responsibility educators, social service personnel, and community members have in alleviating child abuse situations and what support systems are needed.

Bibliography

Anda, R. F., Felitti, V. J., Bremner, J. D., Walker, J. D., Whitfield, C. H., Perry, B. D., . . . Giles, W. H. (2006). The enduring effects of abuse and related adverse experiences in childhood. *European Archives of Psychiatry and Clinical Neuroscience, 256*(3), 174–186.

Bates, E., & Dick, F. (2002). Language, gesture, and the developing brain. *Developmental Psychobiology, 40*(3), 293–310.

Bates, E., Thal, D., & Janowsky, J. S. (1992). Early language development and its neural correlates. In E. S. J. Segalowitz, E. I. Rapin et al. (Eds.), *Handbook of neuropsychology*: 7, 69–110). Amsterdam, The Netherlands.

Belsky, J., Vandell, D. L., Burchinal, M., Clarke-Stewart, K. A., McCartney, K., & Owen, M. T. (2007). Are there long-term effects of early child care? *Child Development, 78*(2), 681–701.

Bremner, J. D., Randall, P., Vermetten, E., Staib, L., Bronen, R. A., Mazure, C., . . . & Charney, D. S. (1997). Magnetic resonance imaging-based measurement of hippocampal volume in posttraumatic stress disorder related to childhood physical and sexual abuse—a preliminary report. *Biological psychiatry, 41*(1), 23-32.

Brown, T. T., & Jernigan, T. L. (2012). Brain development during the preschool years. *Neuropsychology Review, 22*(4), 313–333.

Castellanos, F. X., Lee, P. P., Sharp, W., Jeffries, N. O., Greenstein, D. K., Clasen, L. S., . . . Zijdenbos, A. (2002). Developmental trajectories of brain volume abnormalities in children and adolescents with attention-deficit/hyperactivity disorder. *JAMA, 288*(14), 1740–1748.

Chiron, C., Jambaque, I., Nabbout, R., Lounes, R., Syrota, A., & Dulac, O. (1997). The right brain hemisphere is dominant in human infants. *Brain, 120*(6), 1057–1065.

Chugani, H. T. (1999). PET scanning studies of human brain development and plasticity. *Developmental Neuropsychology, 16*(3), 379–381.

Chugani, H. T., Phelps, M. E., & Mazziotta, J. C. (2008). Positron emission tomography study of human brain functional development. In M. H. Johnson, Y. Munakata, & R. O. Gilmore (Eds.), *Brain development and cognition: A reader* (pp. 101–116). Hoboken: John Wiley & Sons.

Connolly, K., Brown, K., & Bassett, E. (1968). Developmental changes in some components of a motor skill. *British Journal of Psychology, 59*, 305–314.

DeBellis, M. D., Keshaven, M. S., Clark, D. B., Casey, B. J., Giedd, J. B., Boring, A. M., Feresbace, K., & Ryan, N. D. (1999). Developmental traumatology, Part 2: Brain development. *Biological Psychiatry, 45*, 1271–1284.

Denckla, M. B. (1974). Development of motor co-ordination in normal children. *Developmental Medical Child Neurology, 16*, 729–741.

Eliot, L. (1999). *What's going on in there? How the brain and mind develop in the first five-years of life*. New York: Bantam.

Faraone, S.V., & Biederman, J. (1998). Neurobiology of attention-deficit hyperactivity disorder. *Biological Psychiatry, 44*(10), 951–958.

Fletcher, K. L. (2011). Neuropsychology of early childhood. In A. S. Davis (Ed.), *Handbook of pediatric neuropsychology* (pp. 31–36). New York: Springer.

Ford, J. D., Racusin, R., Ellis, C. G., Daviss, W. B., Reiser, J., Fleischer, A., & Thomas, J. (2000). Child maltreatment, other trauma exposure, and posttraumatic symptomatology among children with oppositional defiant and attention deficit hyperactivity disorders. *Child Maltreatment, 5*(3), 205–217.

Fox, N. A., Rubin, K. H., Calkins, S. D., Marshall, T. R., Coplan, R. J., Porges, S. W., Long, J. M., & Stewart, S. (1995). Frontal activation asymmetry and social competence at four years of age. *Child Development, 66*(6), 1770–1784.

Fox, N. A., Schmidt, L. A., Calkins, S. D., & Rubin, K. H. (1996). The role of frontal activation in the regulation and dysregulation of social behavior during the preschool years. *Development & Psychopathology, 8*(1), 89–102.

Giedd, J. N., Snell, J. W., Lange, N., Rajapakse, J. C., Casey, B. J., Kozuch, P. L., Vaituzis, A., Vauss, Y., Hamburger, S., Kaysen, D., & Rapoport, J. L. (1996). Quantitative magnetic resonance imaging of human brain development: Ages 4–18. *Cerebral Cortex, 6*(4), 551–559.

Goodman, J. C. (2001, April). The rate and shape of receptive and expressive vocabulary development in infants and toddlers. Paper presented at the *Society for Research in Child Development*, Minneapolis, MN.

Hart, H., & Rubia, K. (2012). Neuroimaging of child abuse: A critical review. *Frontiers in Human Neuroscience, 6*, 52.

Hill, C., Gormley, W., & Adelstein, S. (2012).. Do the short-term effects of a strong preschool program persist? *Center for Research on Children in the United States, Working Paper, 18*, 17.

LaHoste, G. J., Swanson, J., Wigal, S. B., Glabe, C., Wigal, T., King, N., & Kennedy, J. L. (1996). Dopamine D4 receptor gene polymorphism is associated with attention deficit hyperactivity disorder. *Molecular Psychiatry, 1*(2), 121–124.

Liu, D., Sabbagh, M. A., Gehring, W. J., & Wellman, H. M. (2009). Neural correlates of children's theory of mind development. *Child Development, 0*(2), 318–326.

McCrory, E., De Brito, S. A., & Viding, E. (2012). The link between child abuse and psychopathology: A review of neurobiological and genetic research. *Journal of the Royal Society of Medicine, 105*(4), 151–156.

Neville, H., Andersson, A., Bagdade, O., Bell, T., Currin, J., Fanning, J., Klein, S., Lauinger, B., Pakulak, E., Paulsen, D., & Sabourin, L. (2008). Effects of music training on brain and cognitive development in under-privileged 3-to 5-year-old children: Preliminary results. *Learning, Arts, and the Brain: The Dana Consortium Report on Arts and Cognition* (pp. 105–106). New York and Washington, DC: The Dana Foundation.

Nores, M., Belfield, C. R., Barnett, W. S., & Schweinhart, L. (2005). Updating the economic impacts of the High/Scope Perry Preschool program. *Educational Evaluation and Policy Analysis, 27*(3), 245–261.

Ortiz-Mantilla, S., Choe, M. S., Flax, J., Grant, P. E., & Benasich, A. A. (2010). Associations between the size of the amygdala in infancy and language abilities during the preschool years in normally developing children. *Neuroimage, 49*(3), 2791–2799.

Panksepp, J. (1998). Attention deficit hyperactivity disorders, psychostimulants, and intolerance of childhood playfulness: A tragedy in the making? *Current Directions in Psychological Science*, 7(3), 91–98.

Peisner-Feinberg, E. S., Burchinal, M. R., Clifford, R. M., Culkin, M. L., Howes, C., Kagan, S. L., & Yazejian, N. (2001). The relation of preschool child-care quality to children's cognitive and social developmental trajectories through second grade. *Child Development, 72*(5), 1534–1553.

Pellegrini, A., & Bjorklund, D. F. (1996). The place of recess in school: Issues in the role of recess in children's education and development (Introduction to theme issue, J. Johnson, Theme Coordinator). *Journal of Research in Childhood Education, 11*(1), 5–13.

Perry, B. D. (1996). Incubated in terror: Neurodevelopmental factors in the 'cycle of violence.' In J. D. Osofsky (Ed.), *Children, youth and violence: Searching for solutions* (pp. 2–20). New York: Guilford.

Reynolds, A. J., Magnuson, K. A., & Ou, S. R. (2010). Preschool-to-third grade programs and practices: A review of research. *Children and Youth Services Review, 32*(8), 1121–1131.

Rueda, M. R., Rothbart, M. K., McCandliss, B. D., Saccomanno, L., & Posner, M. I. (2005). *Training, maturation, and genetic influences on the development of executive attention.* Retrieved from www.pries.org/cgr/10.1073/prias.0506897102.

Schweinhart, L. J. (1993). *Significant benefits: The High/Scope Perry Preschool study through age 27* (Monographs of the High/Scope Educational Research Foundation, No. 10). Ypsilanti, MI: High/Scope Educational Research Foundation.

Shankle, W., Landing, B., Rafii, M., Schiano, A., Chen, J., & Hara, J. (1998, March 21). Evidence for a postnatal doubling of neuron number in the developing human cerebral cortex between 15 months and 6 years. *Journal of Theoretical Biology, 191*, 115–140.

Sonuga-Barke, D. J., Dalen, L., & Remington, B. (2003). Do executive deficits and delay aversion make independent contributions to preschool attention-deficit/hyperactivity disorder symptoms? *Journal of the American Academy of Child & Adolescent Psychiatry, 42*(11), 1335–1342.

Tan, A. A., & Molfese, D. L. (2009). ERP correlates of noun and verb processing in preschool-age children. *Biological Psychology, 80*(1), 46–51.

te Nijenhuis, J., Jongeneel-Grimen, B., & Kirkegaard, E. O. (2014). Are headstart gains on the g factor? A meta-analysis. *Intelligence, 46*, 209–215.

Thompson, R. A., & Nelson, C. A. (2001). Developmental science and the media: Early brain development. *American Psychologist, 56*(1), 5–15.

Yoshinaga-Itano, C., Baca, R. L., & Sedey, A. L. (2010). Describing the trajectory of language development in the presence of severe to profound hearing loss: A closer look at children with cochlear implants versus hearing aids. *Otology & Neurotology: Official*

Publication of the American Otological Society, American Neurotology Society [and] European Academy of Otology and Neurotology, *31*(8), 1268.

Zigler, E. F., & Bishop-Josef, S. J. (2006). The cognitive child versus the whole child: Lessons from 40 years of Head Start. In D. G. Singer, R. M. Golinkoff, & K. Hirsh-Pasek (Eds.), *Play = learning: How play motivates and enhances children's cognitive and social-emotional growth* (pp. 15–35). New York: Oxford University Press.

Zigler, E., Gilliam, W. S., & Barnett, W. S. (2011). *The pre-K debates: Current controversies and issues*. Baltimore, MD: Brookes Publishing Company.

6

BRAIN DEVELOPMENT AND LEARNING IN THE ELEMENTARY YEARS

Case 1 The Havenbrook Twins

Both Mr. Sanchez and Mrs. Solomon teach third grade. Mr. Sanchez has enjoyed having Emily, one of the Havenbrook twins in his class, especially because he has observed how much academic growth she has achieved over the year. Emily is a quiet, serious worker who listens carefully to directions, plans work tasks well, asks thoughtful questions, and never disobeys the rules. He believes her executive functioning skills are developing really well. He can always call on her to be the leader of an activity or to help another student who is struggling. His only concern is that she is rather solitary and has only one good friend in the class, but their relationship seems to be beneficial for both of them. Her (non-identical) twin sister, Ellen, is in Mrs. Solomon's class across the hall, and she is also doing well in third grade. In contrast to Emily, however, Ellen is very outgoing and has many friends. Her happy personality is reflected in the way she enjoys learning activities that involve constructing models of nature environments, playing math games, and giving oral reports on science projects. Her teacher is aware of Emily's many talents and involves her in leadership roles because she is very popular with the other children. In fact, she might be called a classroom "star"! On the other hand, Emily's creative nature causes her to be "flighty" and Mrs. Solomon has to remind her to use her executive functioning skills more deliberately. The twins' parents have noted that since their birth, the twins have very different personalities and they sometimes juggle their parenting skills to meet the needs of both girls. However, they are pleased that both girls are very successful in school.

Case 2 Kenny's Reading Problem

When Kenny, age 10, was in fourth grade, his teacher noticed that he was having difficulty reading the grade-level material, especially in comprehending chapter books. He had no behavior problems and had strong relationships with his friends and family, however. He had a great deal of energy, a contagious amount of enthusiasm, and a positive outlook on life. He was especially good at problem-solving in math class, was active in student activities, and enjoyed athletics. However, he had a hard time making sense out of stories that seemed easy for everyone else and said that reading had always been "a little hard" for him. Kenny's parents agreed with the teacher's concerns, noting that from third grade on, he had difficulty with reading. Kenny's father, an accountant, said he did not want his son to "hate reading" in school the way he (the father) had. Kenny's birth history and developmental milestones were typical but he did have Tympanostomy tubes in his ears because of chronic earaches. Kenny's mother remembered he had difficulty learning letters, writing them backward, and trouble in rhyming. A comprehensive evaluation showed Kenny had a learning disability in reading, although he was cognitively above average with many strengths. Weaknesses were in phonological processing, word reading, reading fluency, verbal reasoning, and reading comprehension. He received an individualized education program (IEP) recommending multisensory reading interventions for phonological skills and use of computer programs to increase reading fluency and comprehension. In a later meeting, the multidisciplinary team noted his reading fluency had improved but his comprehension still lagged. They decided to continue the plan and add a discussion-based reading comprehension program, and Kenny responded well to this. Now Kenny is a fifth grader and beginning to read more challenging material using techniques he has been taught. He reads chapter books about sports and fantasy such as "Harry Potter."

Review of Brain Development During the Elementary Years

Although there has not been extensive research focused on the anatomical brain development of children older than 6, synaptogenesis, as measured by glucose metabolic rates, continues to occur throughout the 6 to 8 age period (Chugani, 1999). Synaptic density in the frontal lobe peaks at about 7 years, as compared with peaking at 1 year in the visual cortex (Eliot, 1999). Recent longitudinal studies of children's brain development have given information about both the elementary child's brain development and older age level aspects of brain development (see Gogtay et al., 2004; Lebel & Beaulieu, 2011; Toga, Thompson, & Sowell, 2006). During the elementary age period, brain development is accompanied by growth in motor coordination, metalinguistic awareness, self-efficacy knowledge, and social competence. According to Bauer and colleagues (2011), some gender differences in brain development also have been noted, such as the hippocampus being larger in girls and the amygdala being larger in boys, but they suggest that further research is needed to determine how such differences are related to children's behavior.

Although at age 4 brain glucose use is twice that of adults, it gradually declines through early and middle childhood and adolescence as the pruning process occurs (Chugani et al., 1993). However, children of 7 to 14 still activate a larger brain area than adults use when carrying out discrimination tasks (Haier et al., 1992). The levels of dopamine, a neurotransmitter that affects brain circuits, rise only gradually in the frontal lobe, and myelination of the frontal lobe continues until early adulthood. The slow maturation of the frontal lobe improves cognitive abilities and some abilities seem to mature earlier than others. For example, there are advances in the speed and efficiency of memory and intellectual processes such as problem-solving. By the age of 6, individual child brain differences already may be relatively stable. Researchers have reported that differences in children's brain organization are reflected in such skills as phonological awareness, extensiveness of vocabulary, and/or later reading and math abilities (Molfese et al., 1999; Fletcher et al., 1994). Studies using measures of electrical transmission within the brain (ERPs) indicate that the pruning of superfluous neural circuits proceeds during the elementary age years. Children's observation and reaction times grow shorter and their performance on cognitive tests grows faster. Most studies show the largest gains in speed between ages 5 and 11 (Fry & Hale, 2000). Speed of processing, related to the P300 wave, which is related to being conscious of mental experiences, does not show up unambiguously until age 4 or 5 and does not reach full amplitude and speed until adolescence (Eliot, 1999). By age 6 or 7, children begin to achieve adult-level performance on tasks requiring attention and inhibition of impulses, but they must put greater effort into such tasks. According to Pfueller and colleagues (2011), who investigated the P300 wave in children age 6 to 18 as they responded to the "oddball paradigm," an age-dependent effect of habituation (the decrease in response to stimuli after repeated exposure), the P300 amplitude increased in younger children but there was no significant change for adolescents. They concluded that younger children activate a larger neuronal pool and must exclude unnecessary neurons during their short-term learning.

Schooling appears to affect memory skills and cognitive development, perhaps because children develop "meta" strategies that enable them to think about their learning abilities and to channel their learning (Alloway et al., 2004; Kail, 1998, 2003). Children's memories also improve because they learn to apply memory strategies that enable the brain's memory functions to be more efficient. ERP studies of children's processing speed have shown that their reaction and inspection times grow shorter and performance on cognitive tests grows faster as their age increases. The largest gains in speed occur between ages 5 and 11 (Hale, 1990). Children of age 6 or 7 begin to achieve adult levels of performance on tasks requiring attention and inhibition of impulses, and evidence of this is from studies showing their P300 wave responses increase rapidly (McIsaac & Polick, 1992). These brain wave changes occur at the same time in which Piaget (1952) noted that children were reaching the stage of concrete operational thought, in which they demonstrate logical reasoning about conservation of matter (e.g., quantities, length, weight). This congruence suggests that theoretical relationships about cognitive processing growth are linked to brain development processes.

Fischer (Fischer & Rose, 1998; Fischer, 2008) has related neo-Piagetian theory of levels of cognitive development to emerging evidence on dynamic system cortical growth cycles. Fischer describes four nested cognitive developmental cycles or levels: reflexes (3 to 11 weeks), actions (3–4 months to 11–13 months), representations (2 years to 7 years), and abstractions (10 years to 20 years). Within each cycle, there are three tiers: *single* competencies develop, then *mappings* of these competencies, and finally, they become competency *systems*. Fischer and Rose state that there are "parallels of these cortical cycles with the cognitive developmental cycles for levels and tiers" (p. 58). Both Fischer and Thatcher (Thatcher, 1994; Thatcher et al., 2005) describe systematic spurts in cognition at certain age periods, indicating these cycles of cognitive development follow a definite re-organizational pattern in the brain. In an analysis of EEG studies of arithmetic performance, Fischer suggested that cortical growth spurts reflect the emergence of new skills, and he notes that the prefrontal cortex is the source of cognitive changes. He indicates that there are implications for educators but cautions that more direct evidence is needed because "the current state of knowledge does not allow direct extrapolation from brain growth cycles to educational practice" (Fischer & Rose, 1998, p. 146).

This age period involves more individualization of brain structures and functions as children interact with a wider level of environmental experiences. Although elementary-age children can overcome some types of dire early childhood circumstances, by the end of this age period, human opportunities for significant expansion of the synaptic system do appear to be limited. This age period also involves refinements in the brain's wiring system, including dendritic, synaptic, and myelination increases, and these processes are greatly influenced by the experiential environment of children. Often learning disabilities and attention deficit disorders are diagnosed. In the past, most evidence for these problems and the hypotheses relating them to brain functioning came from neuropsychological evaluations by psychologists rather than from brain imaging research. However, a large body of research on these issues is now coming from MRI and other brain imaging research and from ERP studies.

Taylor, Khan, and Malone (1999) studied the development of attentional processes in children age 7 to 12 using two types of tasks and found that there were decreases in P3 latency with age, task, and an age by task interaction. That is, the time it took children to respond to the stimuli presented was shorter as they grew older. Sussman and Steinschneider (2011) noted differences in MMN, P3b, and N2b responses of younger and older elementary age children who watched a video with loudness and pitch changes; they found younger children's brains processed loudness and pitch changes differently, but 10- to 12-year-olds processed loudness and pitch similarly. Henderson et al. (2011) investigated brain wave patterns in children 8 to 10 when they observed congruent and incongruent picture–word pairs and found their peak amplitude of the ERP waveform (highest activity level) was more negative for semantically incongruent picture–word pairs than for congruent picture–word pairs, indicating their brains distinguished between congruent and incongruent stimuli. In a study of executive functioning, Rueda and colleagues (2005) found that both the anterior cingulate and lateral prefrontal areas were involved in this process, with children who were trained able to do better on the tasks. In a review of brain imaging studies focused on attentional network circuitry, Fernandez-Duque, Baird, and Posner (2000) concluded that maturation and learning both influenced how children's mid-frontal brain areas reacted in attention studies, especially those involving conflict resolution, error correction, and emotional regulation.

Jonkman (2006) compared the speed of processing (P300) and executive functioning at different age levels (ratio of RT and P300 latency divided by accuracy) and found that these waves were absent in the younger subjects and reached maturity in early adulthood. In a face-recognition memory task, Itier and Taylor (2004) found that children age 8 to 16 showed larger amplitudes in P1 and N170 for repeated stimuli and developmental progress in face processing ability. Also, a longitudinal study of cognitive control ability (Lamm, Zelazo, & Lewis, 2006) found the frontal N2 latencies component of the ERP, used as an index of cognitive control, decreased with age, with the cingulate cortex and orbitofrontal cortex generating greatest amplitudes. The researchers concluded that decreases in N2 amplitude but not latencies reflected development of cognitive control.

Studies of brain activation during typical children's performance on academically related tasks also have been of interest. One longitudinal study of phonological processing during rhyming indicated that different aspects of phonological processing rely on different neural systems (Grossi et al., 2001). The researchers reported that although the negative slow wave to primes that is larger over left anterior regions in adult studies was present in children, frontal asymmetry to primes increased with age and correlated with reading and spelling scores. Coch and colleagues (2005) looked at non-word rhyming developmental effects and found that even over the short age period from 6 to 8, the ERPs elicited by the primes changed, with beginning readers showing N1 enhancement to alliterating word and non-word targets that differed from preschool and older reader responses. In an ERP study of number knowledge researchers found that second grade children were already showing a response similar to adults but younger children drew upon distinct ERP processes to perform the tasks, reflecting the development of functional specialization of the parietal cortex (Gebuis et al., 2009).

A recent area of research is whether video games activate brain areas differently at various ages. Two pilot studies investigating ERP patterns of children age 6 to 11 obtained during play with video games (Bergen et al., 2017; Schroer et al., 2016) involved comparing games that required either "right/wrong" answers or "creative" answers. A third study investigated brain wave elicitation in a spatial learning task. Although these studies suggest differences in children's brain activation when they are playing video games that call on varied skills, further study is needed to probe the implications related to effects of video game play on long-term brain development.

Impact of Genetic/Environmental Interactions During the Elementary Age Years

Typically, learning disabilities (especially dyslexia, the impairment of ability to read) and various cognitive and social-emotional problem behaviors such as defiance, aggression, and shyness are diagnosed during this age period, even though precursor conditions may have been evident earlier. When children enter formal education, the difficulties they have in learning are usually recognized and referred for remediation. Researchers report that observed phonological awareness and vocabulary richness at kindergarten age predicted long-term school performance in reading and math (Berninger & Richards, 2002, Molfese, Molfese, & Espy, 1999). Hart and Risley (1995) observed that vocabulary differences, even at age 2 years, predicted verbal IQ and language differences at 5 years, and Morrison and colleagues (1997) found that vocabulary at 5 years predicted third grade reading and math scores. Fletcher and colleagues (1994) reported that phonological decoding deficits at 5 years characterize poor readers regardless of IQ or IQ achievement discrepancy and predict persistent reading problems relative to good readers.

ERP studies have helped researchers understand brain functions for children with identified disabilities because the methodology provides "easy access in reliable measures of normal and deviant arousal and state regulation across a wide age range" (Banaschewski & Brandeis, 2007, p. 419). These authors studied links to the attentional allocation, stimulus evaluation, and working memory processes, as well as to processing of language at semantic and syntactic levels by examining the N400 wave in the anterior medial temporal lobe. There also is evidence that dyslexia has a genetic component (Pennington, 1995) because about 40% of dyslexic children have parents and/or siblings with the syndrome. Early fMRI findings by Shaywitz and colleagues (1996) show differing activation patterns in the brain during performance of phonological tasks between these groups. There also may be differences in the cortical vision systems (Eden et al., 1996). Zeffiro and Eden (2000) report that neuroimaging studies of reading and early sensory processing implicate sites in the left hemisphere (e.g., occipitotemporal sulcus, posterior-superior temporal gyrus, inferior parietal cortex). While these are early findings, evidence suggests that "dyslexia is a complex, multifaceted, brain-based disorder . . . that . . . is not reducible to a mere discrepancy between ability and achievement" (Meyer, 2000, p. 325).

Stevens et al. (2013) examined attentional neural mechanisms of kindergarten children who were at risk for reading disabilities and found the group, given supplemental instruction, showed improvement on a literacy measure. ERP results indicated that at the beginning of kindergarten, this group had sensorineural processing delays in comparison to the control group; but following the intervention, this difference was not present, indicating literacy interventions could help. However, another study of children at risk and not at risk for dyslexia that compared children on visual activity for print at kindergarten age, and again in second grade, found continuing differences (Brem et al., 2010). Researchers reported that by second grade, dyslexic children showed differences in the inferior occipitotemporal cortex and left lateralization was reduced as compared to controls. They concluded that children who have a delay in initial visual tuning for print may have reading problems, even after initial reading training. A longitudinal study by Molfese, Molfese, and Modgline (2001), which compared newborn ERP hemispheric measures with the children's intellectual, language, reading, and environmental measures at second grade, found that infant ERP scores and preschool language scores contributed most to variance in second-grade reading scores. That is, auditory variation in newborns' ERP records discriminated the reading performance of the children 8 years later. Such longitudinal ERP studies that compare newborn or preschool brain functioning with developmental difficulty at later ages may be useful in promoting successful interventions at earlier ages. As with findings on brain-autism relationships in the early years, there presently is a lack of longitudinal imaging studies of brain development primarily focused on children who might be at risk for learning disabilities.

Just as children's unique neurocognitive makeup has an impact on academic performance, so too will it affect social cognitive abilities (Perret-Clermont, 1980; Vygotsky, 1967, 1980). Social skills and abilities are part of the cultural-educational world children and teens experience. Difficulties within this domain can range from normal yet potentially difficult adjustments in childhood (such as shyness, being too socially gregarious, manipulative, having friendship difficulties) and can also include genetic disorders that feature social problems (Campbell et al., 2015; Woodin et al., 2001). Just as it is prudent to study and develop treatments for academic skill disabilities, so too should brain-behavior bases for social cognitive difficulties or minor social adjustments experienced in typical development be studied (Baron-Cohen, 1988, Blakemore & Choudhury, 2006; Meyer et al., 2015; Saxe, 2006). There are major differences between children who are normally developing but quiet, shy, and introverted and children who have significant social cognitive concerns involving social distance, nonliteral language understanding, reading emotions, impulsivity, and executive functioning issues.

Suggestions for Fostering Brain Development and Learning

Although brain development at this age is gaining research focus, suggestions for fostering brain development are still speculative. Authors and consumer product developers often stress the importance of brain/cognition relationships but give educational suggestions that are not based on research evidence, and they are not recommended.

For Families

- Families who have positive, emotionally safe environments and high-quality educational experiences at home and school are important at this age also. Negative effects on brain development of extremely poor environments have been documented at this age.
- If families have children with disabilities, they should strongly advocate for help from professionals who know the latest information in brain research, because techniques to support brain efficiency are being developed regularly.
- Research on relationships between early phonological and vocabulary skills and later risks for learning disabilities suggests that parents should actively foster language abilities, including phonological awareness and vocabulary development. Accurate diagnosis and intervention for children with delays should be made by age 7 rather than using a "wait and see" approach.
- If a child is having social issues or concerns, meetings with school personnel (counselor, psychologist, principal, teacher) should be scheduled to discuss whether they see problems and what services, counseling groups, or other resources are available.

For Educators

- Educators should work at lower as well as higher levels of children's cognitive functioning and appreciate the plasticity and cyclical nature of cognitive/brain growth. They can help children relearn/rework concepts, provide contextual support for high-level functioning, and not expect normal functioning to be always at optimal level.

- Educators should provide environments with opportunities for exercising social-emotional, physical-sensory-motor, and language-cognition abilities to strengthen synaptic connections. Mastery experiences promote stronger synaptic connections in basic learning areas.
- Educators can encourage individual children to practice their special skills and talents to strengthen the synaptic connections related to these abilities (e.g., artistic, mathematical, literary, scientific).
- Until the pruning process is better understood, educators should help every child develop a plethora of synapses available for pruning, gain strong and rich synaptic connections in areas basic to learning success, and exercise their unique abilities. A curriculum that supports a wide range of abilities, strengths, and learning modes is best.
- Educators should extend the abilities of both boys and girls. Most research shows that while there may be some skill differences in males and females, there is an overlapping range on all dimensions, with many males and females performing similarly. They should avoid gender-stereotyped curriculum approaches.
- Because most educators work in inclusive environments, they should know what brain research suggests for teaching children with disabilities. Research shows the importance of attention to children's vocabulary and phonological deficits, since these relate to reading problems, and should address problems with early numeracy skills (sequencing, number comparison, and quantity understanding).
- Educational experiences should give children opportunities to develop a plethora of synapses, gain strong synaptic connections in areas basic to overall learning success, and exercise their unique abilities. A curriculum that supports many ways to enhance synaptogenesis is best.

For Community Partners and Policy Makers

- Although many communities have strong commitments for funding public elementary schools at high levels, other communities do not provide sufficient funding for schools, either because taxes are low or the tax base is limited. Advocacy groups should inform community leaders and residents that promoting high levels of brain development in future citizens is crucial and that the quality of schools is related to brain development.
- Public schools should have educational practices that are relevant and effective in promoting learning and brain development for all children, including those with special needs. If there are alternative school options (e.g., private charter or religious schools), these schools should have similar supervision and requirements.

Cases 3 and 4 Social Interactions of Alexis and Tamara

Alexis is a fourth grader who is a voracious reader and who also spends time painting, gardening, and playing with her cat, Mr. Stripey. Her mother says that she is a good cook who likes spending time by herself and is a "real thinker." At school, she is very quiet, does not often answer questions unless called upon, and has just one friend, Lucy, with whom she eats lunch and plays during recess. She does not interact with other students except when she is in a group class activity. Her teacher, Mrs. Ginny, has observed that when she works in a group, she has good ideas, offers witty comments, and gets along well with other children, but often seems to "hold back." Mrs. Ginny said that when Alexis hands in her written work, it is often so insightful, accurate, and stellar that she is sure Alexis has much more to offer than she shows. Despite her efforts to involve Alexis and encourage her to be more social, Alexis does not seem willing to change. Mrs. Ginny talked to the school psychologist, Ms. Salvitti, and asked if there was anything she could do to help her become more outgoing. Ms. Salvitti suggested that she might be just a quiet, thoughtful, and somewhat shy girl who had appropriate but reserved relationships with her peers and adults. She did not suggest any special intervention for Alexis. In contrast, Ms. Salvitti described another girl, Tamara, who was an excellent student in math and science but who had problems with social/pragmatic language skills (i.e., deficits in social cognition). She said that Tamara desperately wanted to have more friends but that her classmates rejected her. When she placed Tamara in a group with other students, she was so eager to be with them that she would be "activated" by getting too physically close, impulsively saying unusual things, or acting in ways that were inappropriate for the situation. She had difficulty understanding the perspectives of other students and often talked to students about topics that were not interesting to them. The others would sometimes just stare at her, and then Tamara would abruptly walk away or recoil into her own seat. Thus, she didn't have any close friends. Tamara also had difficulty understanding nonliteral language and missed the meanings of jokes or sarcasm. Based on her parents' request, Tamara was seen for individual counseling and was then a participant in a social skills group. The counseling focused on having Tamara better understand the social and emotional messages she conveyed. For instance, Ms. Salvitti said that on the playground, Tamara would pursue other students who had already given her social cues that told her to "back off." A big breakthrough, Ms. Salvitti thought, was being able to put her in an enrichment class that had other students who were interested in topics that Tamara liked. Tamara said that she felt "really good" about being able to talk about stuff that she thought about in her own head.

Study Guide/Questions for Discussion

- Discuss how pruning and arborization is reflected in elementary children's social, emotional, and cognitive development. How might the intense focus on preferred experiences at this age affect brain development? Give examples of changes in behavior that reflect pruning and growth dynamics.
- Compare developmental issues that Emily and Ellen are encountering and suggest ways that both their teachers could encourage their development using knowledge of brain development processes and understanding of the personalities and cognitive strengths of each child.
- Kenny, Alexis, and Tamara all are having problems in school. Select one of them and describe developmental challenges they may face in relation to information on optimal brain development during this age period. Give suggestions for educational supports that could enhance that development and foster strong synaptic connections.
- Because of the increased amount of time that children of this age spend using technology-augmented materials, these behaviors may affect the brains' pruning and selective growth processes. Plan a talk on elementary age children's brain development and potential effects of intensive or extensive video game play or electronic social media use. What suggestions would you give about how to optimize these children's brain development?

Bibliography

Alloway, T. P., Gathercole, S. E., Willis, C., & Adams, A. M. (2004). A structural analysis of working memory and related cognitive skills in young children. *Journal of Experimental Child Psychology*, *87*(2), 85–106.

Banaschewski, T., & Brandeis, D. (2007). Annotation: What electrical brain activity tells us about brain function that other techniques cannot tell us—a child psychiatric perspective. *Journal of Child Psychology and Psychiatry*, *48*(5), 415–435.

Baron-Cohen, S. (1988). Social and pragmatic deficits in autism: Cognitive or affective?. *Journal of autism and developmental disorders*, *18*(3), 379-402.

Bauer, P. J., Lukowski, A. F., & Pathman, T. (2011). Neuropsychology of middle childhood development (6 to 11 years old). In A. S. Davis (Ed.), *Handbook of pediatric neuropsychology* (pp. 37–46). New York: Springer.

Bergen, D., Schroer, J., Thomas, R., Zhou, X., Chou, M., & Chou, T. (2017). Child ERP responses to two stimuli types in videogame situations: Study 1 & 2 comparisons. *Journal of Research in Childhood Education, 31*(1), 160–175.

Berninger, V. W., & Richards, T. L. (2002). *Brain literacy for educators and psychologists.* New York: Academic Press.

Blair, C., & Raver, C. C. (2012). Child development in the context of adversity: Experiential canalization of brain and behavior. *American Psychologist, 67*(4), 309.

Brem, S., Bach, S., Kucian, K., Kujala, J. V., Guttorm, T. K., Martin, E., . . . Richardson, U. (2010). Brain sensitivity to print emerges when children learn letter—speech sound correspondences. *Proceedings of the National Academy of Sciences, 107*(17), 7939–7944.

Campbell, L. E., McCabe, K. L., Melville, J. L., Strutt, P. A., & Schall, U. (2015). Social cognition dysfunction in adolescents with 22q11. 2 deletion syndrome (velo-cardio-facial syndrome): Relationship with executive functioning and social competence/functioning. *Journal of Intellectual Disability Research, 59*(9), 845–859.

Chugani, H. T. (1999). PET scanning studies of human brain development and plasticity. *Developmental Neuropsychology, 16*(3), 379–381.

Chugani, H. T., Phelps, M. E., & Massiotta, J. C. (1993). Positron emission tomography study of human brain functional development. In M. H. Johnson (Ed.), *Brain development and cognition: A reader* (pp. 125–143). Oxford, England: Blackwell.

Coch, D., Grossi, G., Skendzel, W., & Neville, H. (2005). ERP Nonword rhyming effects in children and adults. *Journal of Cognitive Neuroscience, 17*(1), 168–182.

Crone, E. A., & Ridderinkhof, K. R. (2011). The developing brain: From theory to neuroimaging and back. *Developmental Cognitive Neuroscience, 1*(2), 101–109.

Eden, G. F., Van Meter, J. W., Rumsey, J. M., Maisog, J. M., Woods, R. P., & Zeffiro, T. A. (1996). Abnormal processing of visual motion in dyslexia as revealed by functional brain imaging. *Nature, 382*, 66–69.

Eliot, L. (1999). *What's going on in there? How the brain and mind develop in the first five-years of life.* New York: Bantam.

Fernandez-Duque, D., Baird, J. A., & Posner, M. I. (2000). Executive attention and metacognitive regulation. *Consciousness and Cognition, 9*(2), 288–307.

Fischer, K. W. (2008). Dynamic cycles of cognitive and brain development: Measuring growth in mind, brain, and education. In A. M. Battro, K. W. Fischer, & P. J. Lena. *The Educated Brain: Essays in Neuroeducation* (pp. 127–150). Cambridge, UK: Cambridge University Press.

Fischer, K. W., & Rose, S. P. (1998, November). Growth cycles of brain and mind. *Educational Leadership*, 56–60.

Fletcher, J. M., Shaywitz, S. E., Shankweiler, D. P., Katz, L., Liberman, I. Y., Stuebing, K. K. Francis, D. J., Fowler, A. E., & Shaywitz, B. (1994). Cognitive profiles of reading disability: Comparisons of discrepancy and low achievement definitions. *Journal of Educational Psychology, 86*(1), 6–23.

Flowers, D. L., Wood, F. B., & Naylor, C. E. (1991). Regional cerebral blood flow correlates of language processes in reading disability. *Archives of Neurology, 48*, 637–643.

Fry, A. F., & Hale, S. (2000). Relationships among processing speed, working memory, and fluid intelligence in children. *Biological Psychology, 54*(1), 1–34.

Gebuis, T., Herfs, I. K., Kenemans, J. L., de Haan, E. H. F., & van der Smagt, M. J. (2009). The development of automated access to symbolic and non-symbolic number knowledge in children: An ERP study. *Cognitive Neuroscience, 30*, 1999–2008.

Gogtay, N., Giedd, J. N., Lusk, L., Hayashi, K. M., Greenstein, D., Vaituzis, A. C., . . . Rapoport, J. L. (2004). Dynamic mapping of human cortical development during childhood through early adulthood. *Proceedings of the National Academy of Sciences of the United States of America, 101*(21), 8174–8179.

Grossi, G., Coch, D., Coffey-Corina, S., Holcomb, P. J., & Neville, H. J. (2001). Phonological processing in visual rhyming: A developmental ERP study. *Journal of Cognitive Neuroscience, 13*(5), 610–625.

Hagerman, R. J., & Polussa, J. (2015). Treatment of the psychiatric problems associated with fragile X syndrome. *Current Opinion in Psychiatry, 28*(2), 107–112.

Hagman, J. O., Wood, F., Buchsbaum, M. S., Tallal, P., Flowers, L., & Katz, W. (1992). Cerebral brain metabolism in adult dyslexic subjects assessed with positron emission tomography during performance of an auditory task. *Archives of Neurology, 49*, 734–739.

Haier, R. J., Siegel, B., Tang, C., Abel, L., & Buchsbaum, M. S. (1992). Intelligence and changes in regional cerebral glucose metabolic rate following learning. *Intelligence, 16*(3), 415–426.

Hale, S. (1990). A global developmental trend in cognitive processing speed. *Child Development, 61*, 653–663.

Hart, B., & Risley, T. R. (1995). *Meaningful differences in the everyday experiences of young American children*. Baltimore, MD: Paul H. Brooks.

Henderson, L. M., Baseler, H. A., Clarke, P. J., Watson, S., & Snowling, M. J. (2011). The N400 effect in children: Relationships with comprehension, vocabulary and decoding. *Brain & Language, 117*(2), 88–99. doi:10.1016/j.bandl.2010.12.003.

Itier, R. J., & Taylor, M. J. (2004). Face recognition memory and configural processing: A developmental ERP study using upright, inverted, and contrast-reversed faces. *Journal of Cognitive Neuroscience, 16*(3), 487–502.

Jonkman, L. M. (2006). The development of preparation, conflict monitoring and inhibition from early childhood to young adulthood; a Go/Nogo ERP study. *Brain Research, 1097*(1), 181–193.

Kail, R. V. (1998). *Children and their development*. Upper Saddle, NJ: Prentice Hall.

Kail, R. V. (2003). Information processing and memory. In M. H. Bornstein, L. Davidson, C. L. M. Keyes, & K. A. Moore (Eds.), *Well-being: Positive development across the life course. Crossroads in contemporary psychology* (pp. 269–279). Mahwah, NJ: Erlbaum.

Lamm, C., Zelazo, P. D., & Lewis, M. D. (2006). Neural correlates of cognitive control in childhood and adolescence: Disentangling the contributions of age and executive function. *Neuropsychologia, 44*, 2139–2148.

Lebel, C., & Beaulieu, C. (2011). Longitudinal development of human brain wiring continues from childhood into adulthood. *The Journal of Neuroscience, 31*(30), 10937–10947.

Liu, D., Sabbagh, M. A., Gehring, W. J., & Wellman, H. M. (2004). Decoupling beliefs from reality in the brain: An ERP study of theory of mind. *NeuroReport, 15*(6), 991–995.

McIsaac, H., & Polick, J. (1992). Comparison of infant and adult P300 from auditory stimuli. *Journal of Experimental Child Psychology, 53*, 115–128.

Meyer, M. L., Taylor, S. E., & Lieberman, M. D. (2015). Social working memory and its distinctive link to social cognitive ability: An fMRI study. *Social Cognitive and Affective Neuroscience, 10*(10), 1338–1347.

Meyer, M. S. (2000). The ability-achievement discrepancy: Does it contribute to an understanding of learning disabilities? *Educational Psychology Review, 12*(3), 315–337.

Molfese, D. L., Molfese, V. J., & Espy, K. A. (1999). The predictive use of event-related potentials in language development and the treatment of language disorders. *Developmental Neuropsychology, 16*(3), 373–377.

Molfese, V. J., Molfese, D. L., & Modgline, A. A. (2001). Newborn and preschool predictors of second-grade reading scores: An evaluation of categorical and continuous scores. *Journal of Learning Disabilities, 34*(6), 545-554.

Morrison, F. J., Albers, D. M., & Griffith, E. M. (1997). Nature-nurture in the classroom: Entrance age, school readiness and learning in children. *Developmental Psychology, 33*(2), 254–262.

Pennington, B. (1995, January). Genetics of learning disabilities. *Journal of Child Neurology, 10*(Suppl 1), S69–S77.

Perret-Clermont, A. N. (1980). *Social interaction and cognitive development in children*. Academic Press.

Perry, B. D. (1996). Incubated in terror: Neurodevelopmental factors in the 'cycle of violence.' In J. D. Osofsky (Ed.), *Children, youth and violence: Searching for solutions* (pp. 2–20). New York: Guilford.

Pfueller, U., Oelkers-Ax, R., Gmehlin, D., Parzer, P., Roesch-Ely, D., Weisbrod, M., & Bender, S. (2011). Maturation of P300 amplitude and short-term learning as reflected by P300 habituation between trial blocks in children. *International Journal of Psychophysiology, 79*(2), 184–194.

Piaget, J. (1952). *The origins of intelligence in children*. New York: International Universities Press.

Rueda, M. R., Rothbart, M. K., McCandliss, B. D., Saccomanno, L., & Posner, M. I. (2005). *Training, maturation, and genetic influences on the development of executive attention*. Retrieved from www.pries.org/cgr/10.1073/prias.0506897102.

Saxe, R. (2006). Uniquely human social cognition. *Current Opinion in Neurobiology, 16*(2), 235–239.

Schroer, J., Bergen, D., Thomas, R., (June, 2016). *Event-Related Potentials of Children Aged 6-12 during Naïve Optics Educational Videogame Play Show Positive Wave Amplitudes at Pz*. Poster presentation at the Association for Psychological Science, Chicago.

Shaywitz, S. E., Fletcher, J. M., & Shaywitz, B. A. (1996). A conceptual model and definition of dyslexia: Findings emerging from the Connecticut Longitudinal Study. In J. H. Beitchman (Ed.), *Language, learning, and behavioral disorders: Developmental, biological and clinical perspectives* (pp. 199–223). New York: Cambridge University Press.

Stevens, C., Harn, B., Chard, D., Currin, J., Parisi, D., & Neville, H. (2011). Examining the role of attention and instruction in at-risk kindergartners: Electrophysiological measures of selective auditory attention before and after an early literacy intervention. *Journal of Learning Disabilities, 46*, 73–86. doi:10.1177/00222.1941141787.

Sussman, E. S., & Steinschneider, M. (2011). Attention modifies sound level detection in young children. *Developmental Cognitive Neuroscience, 1*(3), 351–360. doi:10.1016/j.dcn.2011.01.003.

Taylor, M. J., Khan, S. C., & Malone, M. A. (1999). Parallel and serial attentional processes: A developmental ERP study. *Developmental Neuropsychology, 15*(3), 351–358.

Thatcher, R. W. (1994). Psychopathology of early frontal lobe damage: Dependence on cycles of development. *Development and Psychopathology, 6*(4), 565–596.

Thatcher, R. W., North, D., & Biver, C. (2005). EEG and intelligence: Relations between EEG coherence, EEG phase delay and power. *Clinical Neurophysiology, 116*(9), 2129–2141.

Toga, A. W., Thompson, P. M., & Sowell, E. R. (2006). Mapping brain maturation. *Trends in Neurosciences, 29*(3), 148–159.

Vygotsky, L. S. (1967). Play and its role in the mental development of the child. *Soviet Psychology*, *5*(3), 6–18.
Vygotsky, L. S. (1980). *Mind in society: The development of higher psychological processes*. Cambridge, MA: Harvard University Press.
Wood, F. B., Flowers, D. L., & Buchsbaum, M. S. (1991). Investigation of abnormal left temporal functioning in dyslexia through rCBF, auditory evoked potential responses and positron emission tomography. *Reading and Writing Interdisciplinary Journal*, *4*, 81–95.
Woodin, M., Wang, P. P., Aleman, D., McDonald-McGinn, D., Zackai, E., & Moss, E. (2001). Neuropsychological profile of children and adolescents with the 22q11. 2 microdeletion. *Genetics in Medicine*, *3*(1), 34–39.
Zeffiro, T., & Eden, G. (2000). The neural basis of developmental dyslexia. *Annals of Dyslexia*, *50*(1), 1–30.

7

BRAIN DEVELOPMENT AND LEARNING IN THE MIDDLE CHILDHOOD YEARS

Case 1 Cyan Becomes a Middle Schooler

At age 11, Cyan was at the top of the grade rank (fifth grade) at his elementary school. He was one of the top leaders in the building. However, he then entered the sixth grade and began the middle schooler experience. Typically, these are years when most children experience significant bodily changes, increased desire to spend time with their peers, and heightened emphasis on academic areas that used to be focused upon attaining basic skills. In sixth grade, Cyan was still the same height that he was in fifth grade, and after his first day at middle school, he talked with amazement about how many of the seventh graders, especially the girls, were "amazons." One of his best friends, Ben, grew 7 inches over the summer while Cyan only grew 2 inches. He thought the one craziest thing about his new school was that he had to use his locker between classes that were in very different rooms and halls. Throughout his middle school years, Cyan will probably grow at a steady pace and eventually hit a growth spurt, probably in seventh grade. During his first year of middle school he tried some new sports, played an instrument in the band, and has gotten used to the rhythm of changing classes, having to obey different rules, avoiding detention, keeping up with homework, and having to go to his first dance. As Cyan is now taking more advanced coursework, he is finding out that he is a stronger student in math and science than in history and English. Cyan also is struggling to become better at asking for help, representing himself, and standing up to others when he has difficulty or disagrees with what is being discussed. To be successful in middle school, he needs to use the self-regulation skills that he gained during his elementary years.

Case 2 Kendra's Middle School Problems

Kendra's developmental history shows she had difficulty with motor skills. She was described as "clumsy" (having low muscle tone), and started to crawl and walk much later than is typically expected. In elementary school, she had initial difficulties with social skills and was helped with social language by the school psychologist and speech-language pathologist. She had early difficulties with speech-and-language concepts and problems understanding one-to-one correspondence and early number concepts. She was placed in special education support services while she was in first grade and continued to receive services for children with cognitive disabilities throughout her elementary school years. However, she generally turned her work in on time and did well with basic reading, writing, and math-based assignments. Since entering middle school in sixth grade, her language arts, science, and social studies teachers said she was having difficulty comprehending textbook assignments, organizing research papers, and interpreting fiction. In math, she complained that her assignments were now too hard. The math teacher said that she could do basic addition and multiplication but didn't understand underlying concepts. Though Kendra has always had an intense and nervous style relating to people and everyday events, her parents noted that since she started middle school, she was experiencing times of heightened anxiety. She seemed moody and frustrated and had emotional "meltdowns" that seemed more than what would be expected of a middle school child. She also had sleeping difficulties and was becoming difficult to soothe and calm when she faced problems. She complained about not having friends and not being able to trust the friends that she used to have. A school guidance counselor stated she was "high maintenance" because she demanded much of friends, and her teachers noted concerns about her poor academic performance. Her attitude toward school and teachers was increasingly negative. Kendra complained that she couldn't trust her classmates and the teachers did not believe in her. She asserted that she wasn't learning anything because she had to switch classes all the time and the classwork and homework were too hard to understand.

Review of Brain Development During the Middle School Years

A major brain development activity that begins about age 8 or 9 and continues until the late teens is synaptic pruning. Presumably, synapses that have been less used are eliminated and those that were used most frequently are maintained. However, little is known about how this process occurs. Eliot (1999) has commented,

> It is the prolonged pruning period that fixes the overall quality of that ability, because this is when experience—translated into neural activity—decides which connections will be preserved and, consequently, how the brain will be permanently wired for certain ways of thinking, perceiving, and acting. As long as an excess number of synapses are present, the brain remains maximally plastic and can develop in a variety of ways. But once those excess synapses are gone, the critical period is over, and it must make do with its existing circuitry; there's no trading up for a faster computer.
> *(p. 38)*

While synaptogenesis begins to lessen during this age period, myelination continues actively at least through the first decade, and longer in certain parts of the brain, such as in the area around the parahippocampal gyrus, where there is a doubling in the extent of myelination relative to brain weight (Benes et al., 1994). Glucose rates begin a slow decline beginning around age 9 and reach adult rates by 20 years (Chugani, 1999). Thus, the primary pruning period appears to be about as long as the primary synaptogenesis period.

Speed and efficiency of memory continues to develop during this age period. Nelson and colleagues (2000), who studied spatial working memory in children 8 to 11 years, found that it was localized primarily in the middle frontal gyrus, in the superior frontal gyrus, and in the left cingulate. The children's accuracy of memory was similar to the memory of healthy adults with like activation in the posterior parietal region and dorsal aspects of the frontal cortex. Using electrophysiological markers of cortical change, Travis (1998) looked at speed of processing and executive functioning in children 9 and older and found that there were electrophysiological markers associated with these abilities. Information gained through PET scans during a thumb-to-finger tapping activity showed adults had less activation in the temporal lobe and angular and posterior gyri, and more increase in blood flow in the cerebellum, suggesting that once a routine activity is learned and automated within the brain, the higher brain centers are less involved (Mueller et al., 1998).

As the maturation of the prefrontal cortex continues, critical thinking and problem-solving abilities initially become more evident, and may wax and wane for a time, upon which the regulation of emotional states and judgments greatly improves. It is this waxing and waning of middle childhood that can often give the picture of a pre-teen awkwardly transitioning into higher levels of adolescent judgment and choice-making. Functions such as planning, rehearsing future actions, predicting, and controlling emotion with logical thought (through cortex/limbic system connections) all develop greatly in late childhood, and this maturational process continues through adolescence (Siegel, 2013; Sylwester, 1995). Thompson and Nelson (2001) assert that brain regions most relevant to higher cognition are progressing greatly and research shows "how significantly children develop during this period in their thinking, social functioning, self-control, and other capacities" (p. 10). Bauer and colleagues (2011) caution, however, that although during this period of development children show much progress toward "adult-like patterns of thought," their cognitive abilities "are by no means complete" (p. 38).

Although male and female adult brains seem to show some differences (albeit with a wide overlap between genders), there are still relatively few differences seen in girls' and boys' brain structure and function in middle childhood. However, during this age period there may be a narrowing of interests in some areas and focusing of interests in others, which may occur differentially for girls and boys. For example, although boys and girls perform equally well on mathematics in fourth grade (Price et al., 2013), some girls seem to abandon mathematical interests during this later age period. Similarly, boys who continue to have interests in music and dance or other artistic areas may be ostracized by other boys, and this peer pressure may cause boys to narrow their content interests.

Impact of Genetic/Environmental Interactions During the Middle School Years

The middle school period is also a time when a number of brain-related concerns can emerge, most of which have both a genetic and an environmental component. There are some problems that may occur or become more noticeable during this age period, which are based on children's previous developmental issues, such as cognitive impairments and/or emotional instabilities. Often a child with a mild level of cognitive impairment or emotional problems can function relatively well in elementary school, but when the more demanding curriculum of middle school is presented, these children may show increasing difficulty.

In addition to a more demanding curriculum, middle school is a time of marked change as students have to negotiate lockers, change classrooms, and engage with an increasingly complex social networks of peers. For children with developmental disabilities and their families, this time can be especially daunting (Ashby, 2010; Bolourian & Blacher, 2016; Nansel et al., 2003). The term "developmental disabilities" encompasses moderate to severe disabilities diagnosed in childhood, including intellectual disabilities, and conditions included under that label may vary significantly. They may be related to birth trauma, genetic and chromosomal conditions, exposure to prenatal or perinatal issues, or to postnatal risk factors. Examples of developmental disabilities include fragile X syndrome, Down syndrome, spina bifida, 22q11.2 microdeletion syndrome, Williams syndrome, and fetal alcohol syndrome. Some disabilities are related to birth trauma, others to genetic and chromosomal conditions, and some to exposure to prenatal, perinatal, or postnatal risk factors. Likewise, studies regarding the underlying neurological pattern or markers of each condition will vary (Costanzo et al., 2013; Gothelf et al., 2005; Watemberg et al., 2002; Weisman et al., 2015). Although the results from neuroimaging studies have not always shown a consistent pattern, many have found commonalities. Further research in neurobehavioral genetics will help to disentangle the neuropathophysiology of developmental disabilities. As these patterns become clearer and include experiences of parents, teachers, and educational researchers, better interventions can be developed and tailored to improve such conditions.

Other brain-related problems, such as Tourette's syndrome (TS), often are not evident until the adolescent years begin. Although a child may seem to be developing well, the behaviors associated with Tourette's may become very apparent during the middle school years. Thus, it is typically diagnosed at that time. In Tourette's syndrome, the individual may have many brief and stereotypic movement behaviors and unusual vocalizations (tics) that are difficult for them to control. Although this disorder occurs in a small percentage of elementary age children, it often becomes more evident during the age period of 10 to 14. The motor and vocal tics appear randomly and may change in severity over time. Children with other problems such as attention deficit hyperactivity disorder (ADHD), learning disabilities, or other disruptive behaviors are more likely to have TS, and boys are more prone to TS than girls. There appears to be a genetic factor involved. Research on this syndrome has linked it to possible high structural connectivity between the primary motor and sensory cortices (Fahim et al., 2016) and to possible dysfunction of basal ganglia circuits and hypothalamic-pituitary-adrenal axis, making TS individuals more responsive to stress (Du et al., 2010). Children with TS often have anxiety disorders related to the reduced ability of the basal ganglia to suppress cortical activity. They often are distressed because it is difficult for them to control their unusual behavior. It is also clear, however, that many individuals with TS attest to having unique strengths. One of these has to do with a keen ability to process time (Vicario, 2010). It is always important to consider both the deficits *and* assets individuals with neurodevelopmental disorders present.

Another common brain condition that often occurs during this age period, traumatic brain injury (TBI), is directly tied to environmental conditions. Epidemiological surveys indicate that admissions for TBI include 185 to 230 cases per 100,000 children below age 15. Of these cases, 10–15% involve moderate to severe injury (Klaus, 1995). TBI is most often seen either at an early age (e.g., shaking of infants) or in the age period between 9 and 14 when children are more involved in risk-taking activities (see Langlois, Rutland-Brown, & Wald, 2006). Motor vehicle accidents in which the child is a passenger, pedestrian, or bicyclist are the main cause of TBI for young school age children. Males are almost twice as likely to experience TBI as females (Langlois, Rutland-Brown, & Wald, 2006). As children become more involved in extensive organized sports, their chance of sports-related brain injury increases. Until recently, sports injuries to the head often were not even recognized as serious, but recent research shows that brain trauma may occur from severe or even less severe head injuries that are repeated in the same person.

Children who sustain a TBI may have at least transient cognitive impairments such as deficits in intelligence, memory, processing speed, attention, language, and psychomotor skills. Behavioral consequences include poor impulse control and unmanageability, anxiety, irritability, agitation, confusion, loss of spontaneity, lack of insight, and affective disturbances. Researchers who have followed children with varying degrees of TBI over time have found behavioral changes and emerging behavioral problems to be common (e.g., Rutter et al., 1996). Furthermore, family burden and functioning prior to and after the injury are related to behavioral and cognitive outcomes in the child (e.g., Taylor et al., 1995). Although children usually show a rapid recovery from TBI during the first 6 months, those whose injuries are moderate or severe may continue to exhibit cognitive, behavioral, physical, and sensory symptoms. Furthermore, recovery may never be complete. TBI may affect future development through: (1) changes in course and rate of development, (2) reduction in ultimate level of achievement of skills, (3) loss of previously attained skills, and (4) negative effects on development of new skills (Mira, Tucker, & Tyler, 1992). In addition, when children below age 15 experience one TBI, they are twice as likely to sustain another than are children in general. This may be because they are likely to show impulsiveness, poor judgment and safety awareness, or balance and coordination difficulties resulting from the first injury. Further, they are often at risk for psychosocial stressors such as a change in the family roles after the accident, the loss of a family member, a change in friendships, and loss of independence.

There may be many different cognitive and behavioral outcomes in TBI, depending on the nature of the brain insult itself in combination with multiple other factors (e.g., child age, premorbid behavioral or cognitive weaknesses). For example, a common type of brain injury that occurs during vehicle accidents is called a contre-coup injury. This occurs when a child's head strikes the inside of the car and the brain hits the skull at the point of impact and then bounces back to the opposite side of the skull. There can be contusion or bruising of brain matter on the opposite side of the brain. The rotational forces stretch and tear axons, many of which will be permanently damaged and some of which will die. This is called diffuse axonal injury (DAI). This damage is not localized to one area but may result in bleeding within the brain due to disruption of blood vessels. Swelling may also occur, which disrupts blood flow and compresses brain tissue. Thus, the damage due to such an injury can affect multiple brain regions and functions. Depending upon the extent and focal point of their injuries, children may have fatigue or reduced stamina following TBI, which may be partially due to medication, prolonged hospitalization, and inactivity. Daily activities may require more concentration from such children because of cognitive and motor weaknesses, leading to higher levels of fatigue.

Suggestions for Fostering Brain Development and Learning

Often children do well in elementary school but have difficulties when they encounter a middle school environment that requires more executive functioning skills, such as planning, monitoring behavior, and predicting consequences of actions. They usually are required to make new friends in this environment. Adults with knowledge of the brain developmental issues children face at this age can help them to be effective in this transition to middle school.

For Families

- The middle school years are often difficult for families as they may not understand or have resources to cope with changes in physical, mental, and social aspects that their child is undergoing. Families should be able to call upon resources of teachers, administrators, physicians, and other personnel familiar with this age level.
- Expectations of child behavior may be too lenient if parents have not gradually expected more self-controlled behaviors or may be too hard if parents abruptly change expectations because the child is now in middle school. A good approach is to have gradually increasing expectations that prepare children to use greater executive functioning skills, because these skills are essential for a successful middle school experience.
- If a family feels their child does not have the self-regulation and organizational ability needed for middle school entry, they should discuss this issue with school personnel who can suggest support systems that guide the development of such skills.

- Parents should obtain baseline concussion testing for children who will be playing contact sports. Computerized assessment offered through a physician, sports clinic, or neuropsychologist measures reaction time, working memory, processing speed, and executive function. Early measurements can provide comparisons if a child has a concussion and help in planning a treatment plan.

For Educators

- Educators should be aware that this brain development period involves a reorganization that will result eventually in relatively stable structures and functions. Children at this age level often "wax and wane" between more childlike behaviors and more mature ones. Although it is still unclear exactly how the pruning process occurs and what factors influence the selection of synapses to be pruned, it is likely that educational experiences continue to affect this process.
- Educators should discourage middle school age children from deciding prematurely that certain content areas or activities are "not their thing." Intense focus on only one sport or activity to the exclusion of others may not be beneficial when synaptic pruning is beginning in earnest. Encouragement of a broad range of skills, as well as greater mastery of a few skills, is likely to result in more efficient brain organization. Educators should realize that their support or lack of support for wide areas of skill development may affect the middle schooler's brain organization.
- Although there is no definitive research linking formal operational thought processes to specific brain structure/function development, there are parallels in psychological and neurobiological realms. Educators can assume that pruning, which results in faster and more efficient thought processes, may be reflected in children's ability to think abstractly and hypothetically. An educational focus on metacognitive and memory strategies can assist synaptic connection making in frontal lobe areas.
- Educator attention to narrowing gender specialization should be noted. As interests diverge in some areas differentially for girls and boys, there may be differences in pruning of some brain areas. However, until specifics of the interaction of genetic and environmental factors on brain pruning are better known, educators should encourage non-stereotypic and wide rather than narrow foci of interests for both boys and girls.
- Children with TBI should avoid contact sports, diving, or other activities involving risk for a blow to the head. After TBI, children who return to school will need increased supervision and modifications of physical environments to promote safety. Educators should note that although the children may continue to score at grade level on achievement tests after TBI, this score may not accurately reflect their current functioning because these tests usually require use of overlearned skills. Even if they score well, they may

not be ready to return to regular education or may need special help because they may have difficulty with new learning. TBI often causes children to experience deficits in judgment and reasoning and places them at risk for impulsive, uncharacteristic, or potentially dangerous behaviors, even within "safe" school environments. Their problems with fatigue, stamina, and learning difficulties are not motivation deficits or "laziness." The best intervention for TBI is prevention, including training for families and educators in supervisory practices; modifications of home and school environments; and use of accident prevention strategies. If children experience repeated concussions, injuries may compound learning difficulties, so parent education about dangers of extreme sports is important.

For Community Partners and Policy Makers

- Community partners should be sure sports facilities in schools and communities are well designed and that middle school age children's involvement in activities that could result in TBI are not encouraged. They should support safety education and practices with appropriate levels of funding.
- Community partners should continue to support services for children with special needs. Although there is often good community support for special education services for younger children, the middle school environment is a difficult one for all children and thus support for vulnerable children should be of high priority.
- Funding for programs that enable all middle school age children to be well cared for at school and in community should be supported.
- Information on long-term societal effects of TBI, bullying, and other developmental problems that middle school children, especially those with disabilities, often face should be on the agenda of community and national policy makers.

Case 3 Thomas's Brain Trauma

Thomas was an active seventh grader with an impressive record at school. He had never missed a day, and was recognized for all A's in his subjects and for winning a seat in student council. One day, he went to his friend Robby's house where several other boys were jumping on a trampoline. The trampoline had a "cage" made of netting, so Tom thought he would be safe and joined the others as they did daring stunts and aerial displays. He tried to flip by himself and rose very high, but his foot slipped as he began to launch and instead of going straight up, his body went sideways, hit the netting hard, and his head flipped backward and then forward violently and he hit the ground face first. When Robby's mother called 911, an emergency vehicle with paramedics arrived at the scene. Tom was unconscious when brought to the emergency room, where he was treated for a traumatic injury involving a contusion to the frontal area of his head (i.e., a bruise or bleeding on the brain), counter-coup (rapid acceleration and deceleration of the hard surfaces of the head and the soft structures of the brain), and subsequent diffuse axonal injury (shearing or tearing of nerve tissue throughout the brain that often accompanies the experience of counter-coup). Tom regained consciousness within a day and seemed to be aware of who he was and that he was in a hospital, but he also seemed confused and dazed. For the first three weeks in the hospital, he was evaluated and treated by a team of neurologists, nurses, a pediatric neuropsychologist, a speech therapist, a physical therapist, and an occupational therapist. For the last two weeks of his hospital stay, Tom attended a hospital-based school that helped him with transitioning back into his home school. The hospital team and educational professionals from school met and designed an individualized educational plan (IEP) for him that included accommodations. He started school classes but also met with the school counselor, an intervention specialist, and the occupational therapist to continue working on skill areas. After three weeks at home, Tom was feeling better but still had some lingering deficits with attention, choice-making, and reading. He was looking forward to returning to sports soon, and to return to the school student council.

Case 4 Marquivio's "Strange" Behaviors

Marquivio, age 12, is a bright student who gets good grades, enjoys his classes, and likes to spend time with his peers. He has never had any history of behavioral or academic problems. However, his homeroom fifth grade teacher, Mr. Martin, mentioned at a meeting that Marquivio's verbal skills can be both a blessing and a curse for him. He explained, "in class discussions he often talks in a way that shows creativity and a brilliant spark, yet at other times, he says inappropriate and cutting things to teachers and his peers." The principal noted that although he later apologizes and shows genuine remorse for this behavior, Marquivio has told her that he can't always control what he says. Unless he's engaged by something happening in class, it is hard for Marquivio to sit still and work independently for more than a few minutes. He occasionally makes unusual sounds, pops, or movements with his head that some of the other pupils find either amusing or distracting. Because of these behaviors, many students feel uncomfortable around him and aren't sure how to take him. This is hard for Marquivio since he likes to spend time with friends and wants more friendships. Even some of his old friends are not as close as they once were. Mr. Martin began keeping a tally of Marquivio's behaviors so that he could talk to his mother about them. In the call home, Mr. Martin discussed the positive behaviors he shows in class, but then told his mother about his unusual actions. She stated that his parents just had Marquivio evaluated and found out that the problems he was having were due to Tourette's syndrome. He is not intentionally trying to disturb, hurt, or annoy others. She said when he is playing sports, he seems to be able to stop these "tics," but that he is growing reluctant to go to class because he is upset about his behavior and getting anxious that he is going to annoy his teacher or friends. His mother wondered whether Marquivio could take a "time out" by leaving the class briefly when he felt a tic coming on. Mr. Martin agreed but also recommended that the parents meet with him and other school personnel to talk about his situation and how they could help. When Marquivio was diagnosed with Tourette's, the therapist suggested that they contact a representative from a local chapter of the Tourette Association of America (TAA) who would be willing to go with her to a school meeting, and that was arranged.

Study Guide/Questions for Discussion

- Review the information on brain development in middle childhood and identify specific changes that might affect children's social skills, reasoning ability, and physical maturation. Suggest ways that adults might help Cyan, Kendra, and Marquivio to be successful in middle school.
- Think about Thomas and suggest what changes in his school performance in academic, social, or physical development areas might need monitoring. Identify ways his parents and teachers might deal with and accommodate the changes that occur.

- Using information in this chapter, explain how choice-making may be difficult in middle childhood and why a child might seem mature or skillful in one situation but show little signs of progress in another setting.
- Discuss how parents and teachers, armed with knowledge about this age period, should respond to children's behavior. How might their responses be different from the way they would assist adolescents or younger children?
- Review online resources for children with TBI or Tourette's syndrome, including (1) national associations, (2) local chapters, (3) support groups, (4) sample IEPs or 504 reports, (5) books for the student, (6) books for parents and teachers, and (7) software or computer programs available to help them increase such skills as working memory.
- Review school policies regarding athletics and concussions. Identify what school personnel are certified to diagnose and treat concussions. Ask them about definitions they use for baseline testing, concussion, diffuse axonal injury, and policies regarding student athlete repeated concussions. Compare your findings with those in this chapter and with written information.

Bibliography

Ashby, C. (2010). The trouble with normal: The struggle for meaningful access for middle school students with developmental disability labels. *Disability & Society, 25*(3), 345–358.

Bauer, P. J., Lukowski, A. F., & Pathman, T. (2011). Neuropsychology of middle childhood development (6 to 11 years old). In A. S. Davis (Ed.), *Handbook of pediatric neuropsychology* (pp. 37–46). New York: Springer.

Benes, F. M., Turtle, M., Khan, Y., & Farol, P. (1994). Myelination of a key relay zone in the hippocampal formation occurs in the human brain during childhood, adolescence, and adulthood. *Archives of General Psychiatry, 51*(6), 477–484.

Bolourian, Y., & Blacher, J. (2016). Impact of youth with intellectual and developmental disabilities on families: Balancing Perspectives. *Current Developmental Disorders Reports, 3*(2), 1–8.

Chugani, H. T. (1999). PET scanning studies of human brain development and plasticity. *Developmental Neuropsychology, 16*(3), 379–381.

Costanzo, F., Varuzza, C., Menghini, D., Addona, F., Gianesini, T., & Vicari, S. (2013). Executive functions in intellectual disabilities: A comparison between Williams syndrome and Down syndrome. *Research in Developmental Disabilities, 34*(5), 1770–1780.

Du, J. C., Chiu, T. F., Lee, K. M., Wu, H. L., Yang, Y. C., Hsu, S. Y., . . . & Leckman, J. F. (2010). Tourette syndrome in children: an updated review. *Pediatrics & Neonatology, 51*(5), 255-264.

Eliot, L. (1999). *What's going on in there? How the brain and mind develop in the first five-years of life.* New York: Bantam.

Fahim, C., Yoon, U., Das, S., Lyttelton, O., Chen, J., Arnaoutelis, R., . . . & Evans, A. C. (2010). Somatosensory–motor bodily representation cortical thinning in Tourette: effects of tic severity, age and gender. *Cortex, 46*(6), 750-760.

Gothelf, D., Furfaro, J. A., Penniman, L. C., Glover, G. H., & Reiss, A. L. (2005). The contribution of novel brain imaging techniques to understanding the neurobiology of mental retardation and developmental disabilities. *Mental Retardation and Developmental Disabilities Research Reviews, 11*(4), 331–339.

Klaus, J. G. (1995). Epidemiologic features of brain injury in children: Occurrence, children of risk, causes and manner of injury, severity and outcomes. In S. H. Broman & M. E. Michel (Eds.), *Traumatic head injury in children* (pp. 22–39). New York: Oxford.

Langlois, J. A., Rutland-Brown, W., & Wald, M. M. (2006). The epidemiology and impact of traumatic brain injury: A brief overview. *The Journal of Head Trauma Rehabilitation, 21*(5), 375–378.

Mira, M., Tucker, B. F., & Tyler, J. S. (1992). *Traumatic brain injury in children and adolescents: A sourcebook for teachers and other school personnel.* Austin, TX: Pro-Ed.

Mueller, R. A., Rothermel, R. D., Behen, M. E., Muzik, O., Mangner, T. J., & Chugani, H. T. (1998). Developmental changes of cortical and cerebellar motor control: A clinical positron emission tomography study with children and adults. *Journal of Child Neurology, 13*(11), 550–556.

Nansel, T. R., Haynie, D. L., & Simonsmorton, B. G. (2003). The association of bullying and victimization with middle school adjustment. *Journal of Applied School Psychology, 19*(2), 45–61.

Nelson, C. A., Monk, C. S., Lin, J., Carver, L. J., Thomas, K. M., & Truwit, C. L. (2000). Functional neuroanatomy of spatial working memory in children. *Developmental Psychology, 36*(1), 109–116.

Price, G. R., Mazzocco, M. M., & Ansari, D. (2013). Why mental arithmetic counts: Brain activation during single digit arithmetic predicts high school math scores. *The Journal of Neuroscience, 33*(1), 156–163.

Rutter, M., Chadwick, O., Schaffer, D., & Brown, C. (1996). A prospective study of children with head injuries: I. Description and methods. *Psychological Medicine, 10,* 633–645.

Siegel, D. (2013). *Brainstorm: The power and purpose of the teenage brain.* New York: Penguin.

Sylwester, R. (1995). *A celebration of neurons: An educator's guide to the human brain.* Alexandria, VA: Association for Supervision and Curriculum Development.

Taylor, G. H., Drotar, D., Wade, S., Yeates, K., Stancin, T., & Klein, S. (1995). Recovery from traumatic brain injury in children: The importance of the family. In S. H. Broman & M. E. Michel (Eds.), *Traumatic head injury in children* (pp. 188–216). New York: Oxford.

Thompson, R. A., & Nelson, C. A. (2001). Developmental science and the media: Early brain development. *American Psychologist, 56*(1), 5–15.

Travis, F. (1998). Cortical and cognitive development in 4th, 8th, and 12th grade students: The contribution of speed of processing and executive functioning to cognitive development. *Biological Psychology, 48*(1), 37–56.

Tremblay, G. C., & Peterson, L. (1999). Prevention of childhood injury: Clinical and public policy challenges. *Clinical Psychology Review, 19*(4), 415–434.

Vicario, C. M., Martino, D., Spata, F., Defazio, G., Giacchè, R., Martino, V., . . . & Cardona, F. (2010). Time processing in children with Tourette's syndrome. *Brain and Cognition, 73*(1), 28-34.

Watemberg, N., Silver, S., Harel, S., & Lerman-Sagie, T. (2002). Significance of microcephaly among children with developmental disabilities. *Journal of Child Neurology, 17*(2), 117–122.

Weisman, O., Pelphrey, K. A., Leckman, J. F., Feldman, R., Lu, Y., Chong, A., Chen, Y., Monakhov, M., Chew, S. H., & Ebstein, R. P. (2015). The association between 2D: 4D ratio and cognitive empathy is contingent on a common polymorphism in the oxytocin receptor gene (OXTR rs53576). *Psychoneuroendocrinology, 58,* 23-32.

Yeates, K. O., Taylor, H. G., Wade, S. L., Drotar, D., Stancin, T., & Minich, N. (2002). A prospective study of short-and long-term neuropsychological outcomes after traumatic brain injury in children. *Neuropsychology, 16*(4), 514.

Ylvisaker, M., Turkstra, L. S., & Coelho, C. (2005, November). Behavioral and social interventions for individuals with traumatic brain injury: A summary of the research with clinical implications. *Seminars in Speech and Language, 26*(4), 256–267. New York: Thieme Medical Publishers, Inc.

8

BRAIN DEVELOPMENT AND LEARNING IN THE ADOLESCENT YEARS

Case 1 Anita's Adjustment to High School

Anita's parents have felt lucky to have such an attractive and intelligent daughter who thrives on learning, especially because their family background is not known for scholarly success. Though both parents are hard-working, neither went to college, and their cultural ideals have not usually encouraged girls to be scholarly. From a very early age, however, Anita was interested in knowing about everything she encountered, asking questions, coming up with ideas, taking actions that were helpful, and enjoying challenging activities. This type of child is not ever without parental concerns, however, since the parents often have had trouble "keeping up" with Anita's actions and questions. For example, she sometimes contradicted her parents when they made incorrect factual statements and at school she often "read ahead" in the workbooks or did assignments before she was expected to do them. She found books at her grade level boring and wanted higher-level reading options. While these traits sound like evidence of her optimal self-efficacy and cognitive skills, her demonstration of them did not always fit well with home or school tasks. Fortunately, her second-grade teacher recognized her giftedness and her school district had a program for such students, so Anita's elementary school progress was excellent. She coped well with middle school in part because she thrived on being independent and in having some choice of classes. Now that she is in high school, however, she is facing new challenges. In high school, the most popular students are not the smartest ones but the most socially adept and "with it" ones who use social media effectively. When Anita scores at the top of her class on assignments, she is more embarrassed than happy. She has tried to find a friendship group of students more like herself but they have been hard to locate. She is in a lower-income school where few advanced placement classes are offered, so it is difficult for her to meet students like herself in class. She has been bullied at times and rejected from joining groups because other students don't like her "always knowing the answers" and has been the focus of some "mean" remarks on social media. Anita's parents are not wealthy so they don't have the option of sending her to a private school or moving to a suburb with many other high-achieving students. They are trying to save enough to give her a chance to go to college though, because they know she should have that opportunity.

Case 2 Holden's "Laziness" and Homework Issues

Holden's parents and teachers have expressed concerns regarding his academic achievement, motivation, and ability to follow through with work and assignments in school. In middle school, with tutors and parent support, he attained passing grades. However, in high school, his ability to plan, follow through, and complete work satisfactorily had declined. Although in early elementary school, he showed no difficulty acquiring basic academic skills, at times he seemed to lose focus, and he was highly distractible or inattentive when the subject was not of interest. During fifth grade, Holden had a difficult relationship with his teacher and from that time on, he developed increasingly negative emotions about school and struggled more with academics, classwork, and homework completion. This teacher had stated that he was "lazy" and often told Holden that he should "pull himself up by his own bootstraps." In sixth grade, he often "froze" while completing class tests or the state achievement tests. Holden explained that his mind would go blank even when he knew what he wanted to say, and he couldn't write the answer correctly. As a high school student, he has had increasing difficulties with maintaining focus, paying attention, and remembering details. He has a "cavalier attitude," as though he doesn't care about school, and he only occasionally hands in work, which is of inconsistent quality. One of his English teachers, noting his excellent poetry and insightful interpretations in class, commented that "if he would put his mind to it, I think Holden would be one of the best students in class." Holden is physically active, exercises often, and desires to make the school track and baseball teams. He has sleep problems, although he has no usage of alcohol, drugs, or tobacco. As a young child, Holden had chronic ear infections which necessitated the placement of ear tubes. He also was diagnosed with activity-induced asthma and had steroidal treatment. While playing football in the youth league last year, Holden experienced two concussions following helmet-to-helmet contact. Though there was no loss of consciousness, the concussions were noted by the coach and the father of a teammate who was a registered nurse. No follow-up medical treatment was advised by his pediatrician, although he was noted to have severe headaches for a period of a week thereafter.

Review of Adolescent Brain Development

Parents, teachers, and other professionals who have worked with teenagers are familiar with the inconsistency, volatility, and variability that teens often express in their daily lives. The adolescent years often have been defined as a time of "storm and stress," during which many teens experience periods of conflict, moodiness, and strife as they transition from childhood to young adulthood (Compas, Orosan, & Grant, 1993; Hall, 1904; Spear, 2000). Recently, Casey and Jones (2010) discussed new insights gained from studies of human neuroimaging and genetics to help explain "the highly variable stress and turmoil experienced in adolescence" (p. 225). Although adolescence has been recognized as a period of rapid change involving the physical maturation of the body, recent research has shown that it is also a period of rapid changes in the brain. Steinberg (2010) has stated, "the fact that there are changes in the brain during adolescence is no longer debatable" (p. 2). Neuroimaging studies (Arain et al., 2013; Khundrakpam et al., 2016; Giedd, 2008; Giedd & Denker, 2015) reveal that there are massive changes to the brain's hardwiring during the years between age 12 and 25. Such changes may lead to heightened emotions, shifting social relationships, greater autonomy, independence, and conflicting social behaviors, making this period potentially turbulent for teens and for adults who interact with them. These changes not only are extensive but they tend to occur for individuals roughly within the same time period. However, most teens are resilient enough to emerge from this flurry of change and transition and become well-adjusted and competent adults (Offer et al., 1988). The notion that adolescents can express increasing competencies, strengths, and capabilities as they grow also has led to a more optimistic view of this age period rather than considering it as one of just storm and stress (Hines & Paulson, 2006; Lerner et al., 2009; Montemayor, 1983).

In the past, when researchers and physicians discovered that the brain has already reached about 90% of its total volume by age 6, they surmised that the brain was mostly formed or fully developed by the end of childhood. Now it is known that even though the size of the brain doesn't increase much between childhood and the end of adolescence, the brain's wiring becomes ever more complex, efficient, and effective at transmitting and receiving information. The brain produces a large number, even an overabundance, of neural connections just before puberty (Sisk & Foster, 2004). Many of these connections will be effective and used often by the adolescent. However, during this period the brain also removes connections that are not being used through the "use-it-or-lose-it" process of synaptic pruning. Like an advanced computer, the maturing brain develops circuitry or neural networks that can perform several tasks at one time in a manner that heightens efficiency and response time. As the neurons and axons making up these networks mature, the process of myelination (deposit of the special layer of a fatty substance) continues and acts as a neural lubricant that speeds up communication with other neurons. MRI studies of brain development in children and adolescents show increasing white matter (WM) volume over this entire age period. Gray matter (GM) volume, however, peaks at different times in various areas of the brain (Bray et al., 2015; Giedd & Rapoport, 2010). For example, while it is at high density in sensorimotor areas in young children, it is at its highest density in the dorsolateral prefrontal cortex areas during late adolescence. Pruning of such areas thus occurs later in adolescence. According to Bronk (2011), these changes in the adolescent brain "coincide with the end of the critical period for new language acquisition" (p. 49). This appears to be related to diminished white matter growth in the temporal and parietal lobes, areas involved in language, spatial, and auditory functions.

During adolescence, much brain pruning and reorganization is evident in the frontal lobe, which is that part of the brain thought to distinguish humans from other mammals. The prefrontal cortex (PFC) is one of the last regions of the brain to develop fully and connect to other parts of the prefrontal region as well as to the limbic subcortical area. The PFC is the seat of activity often referred to as the "CEO" or executive of the brain that is thought to regulate one's ability to make choices, solve problems, set goals, organize plans, control attention, hold back impulses, regulate emotional reactivity, actively work on new information, and evaluate one's own performance or behavior. As the PFC is pruned, it gives rise to greater cognitive control capacity, higher-order thought, and reasoning skills encountered in adolescence (Yurgelun-Todd, 2007). Though the PFC begins to be activated in adolescence, it is not yet fully active, and because of this brain connections may be routed to different areas until the PFC is fully developed. One key fMRI study (Baird et a1., 1999) found that when identifying strong emotions expressed on faces, teenagers' responses triggered neural activity in the amygdala, which is the area of the brain used to immediately process emotions such as fear, threat, and danger. In contrast, the adults in the study activated their PFC when threatened, suggesting that they had more executive function control, and thus could perform better and more accurately on identifying and dealing with threat. Thus, the ability to make sound judgments when confronted by complex situations, the capacity to control impulses and regulate emotional reactivity, the ability to inhibit the tendency to respond, and the ability to plan effectively all develop during adolescence (Sowell et al., 1999). Recent studies have demonstrated that the ventrolateral prefrontal and anterior cingulate cortices differ in morphology and function, and adolescents engage those structures less than adults do when they are making decisions (Eshel et al., 2007).

Adolescent social cognition, in particular, is greatly affected by amygdala development, and social ostracism can affect its development (Sebastian et al. (2009, 2010). Other areas involved in social cognition include the anterior cingulate cortex, inferior frontal gyrus, and insula, and, according to these researchers, "these areas may be more active and less selective during adolescence than at other points during the lifespan" (p. 137). According to Churchwell and Yurgelun-Todd (2013), because the insula plays a role in prospective thinking, regulation of impulsivity, and anticipation of rewards and losses, as decreases in the cortical thickness of the insula occur, there are also related increases in adolescent ability to have a future orientation and planning ability.

Steinberg (2005) has asserted that although there are beginning to be studies describing changes occurring in the structure of the teenage brain, there is still little research tying those structural changes to functional implications, outcomes, or consequences. Brain development changes often cause adolescents to vacillate from being highly competent with *some* skills to being unable to exert control over *any* such abilities. This imbalanced behavior, choice-making, emotional reactivity, and/or follow-through may reflect the changing and nonlinear structure of the brain, and such variability is a part of the developmental process during these years. Often adolescents may show excellent cognitive and social skills, but may be incapable of making prudent decisions. They can be scattered or haphazard in their ability to solve problems or follow through upon even simple life situations. Thus, they may not be "lazy" but just are still in the process of developing (Gilmore & Boulton-Lewis, 2009; Levine, 2003) and may require specific help, behavioral direction, and understanding to foster their growth.

Impact of Genetic/Environmental Interactions During the High School Years

Because environmental expectations for behavior at this age may not match genetic aspects of brain maturation, there are problems that can occur during this developmental process. For example, one problem in this age period is a tendency for teenagers to engage in risky behaviors that deliver an immediate thrill or highly charged experience. In adolescence, these types of novel experiences are highly desired by teens because they seem to be "wired" to seek out new sensations. This desire to find new experiences is both a blessing and a curse. By seeking out these experiences, teens may gain the ability to make positive social decisions and encounter growth-producing changes. Alternatively, if the adolescent peer group or cultural group is prone to engage in such highly charged novel experiences, they may become involved in potentially risky, dangerous, and even illegal activities. Crews, He, and Hodge (2007) report that, because of these various brain development processes, adolescent decision-making processes may contribute to some teens becoming addicted to drugs, alcohol, and other mind-altering substances. How adolescents will respond to the opportunity to engage in such behaviors may depend upon various factors, including the absence, presence, and responsible quality of their peers; how well they have learned to understand cause-and-effect relationships; how clear they are about consequences that result from their actions; and how motivated they are to explore new interests independently, with or without parental consent. Unfortunately, these behaviors may require the mature development of some brain areas that are just in process. Thus, because executive functioning abilities still are being developed and a lack of judgment or inconsideration of risks can be problematic at this age level, genetic/environmental interactions may result in problematic situations for many adolescents. Giedd and Rapoport (2010) have stated that "appreciating the interplay between limbic and cognitive systems is imperative for understanding decision making during adolescence" (p. 732).

One area that can be problematic for teens is finding a social group that supports and encourages their development. Because of the varied trajectory of individual development, high school usually involves making a new group of friends. Friends from middle school may go elsewhere or change in various ways (either on a slower or faster developmental track) and usually high school has students from many areas who were unknown to the middle schooler. Because of the late-developing brain areas related to social cognition, adolescence is the prime age period in which social rejection or exclusion can be extremely painful and difficult to endure. Indeed, Sebastian and colleagues (2010) note that the brain areas involved in social cognition that are not yet at a mature stage include the medial prefrontal cortex (mPFC), anterior cingulate cortex (ACC), inferior frontal gyrus, posterior-superior temporal sulcus (PSTS), temporo-parietal junction (TPI0), amygdala, and anterior insula. They assert that there can be possible effects of social ostracism in adolescence that may affect long-term development of the social brain. Effects of peer pressure may be subtle or extreme during this age period and, even if subtle, may affect brain development. This sensitivity to peer pressure was explored by Sherman and colleagues (2016), who conducted a social network "likes" study and found that teens were significantly more inclined to "like" photos they thought other teens had liked. The researchers noted that activity in the nucleus accumbens, part of the reward circuitry of the brain, as well as in the prefrontal cortex, increased when the teen's number of "likes" increased. Activity in the dorsal anterior cingulate cortex, a cognitive-control region, was lower when the likes were related to risky activity pictures, but that still activated the adolescent's reward centers, suggesting that self-control and reward responses may be inversely related during this age period. Urosevic and colleagues (2012) note that there are individual differences in the reward-processing areas of the brain that might be related to sensitive periods, such as greater density of synapses in a period of exposure to new environmental rewards, or these differences may be due to different patterns of pruning during this period.

Often depression and other behavioral problems such as eating disorders can occur during adolescence, sometimes related to social relationships but also due to other unresolved issues in the adolescent's life. Such disorders are especially prevalent among adolescent girls. In a study of teens with anorexia nervosa (self-starvation and excessive weight loss), researchers found that, compared to a control group, the anorectic group had lower glucose metabolism in cortical regions (hypometabolism), especially in the frontal and parietal cortices (Delvenne et al., 1995). The researchers hypothesized that the difference might be due to this condition or to associated conditions such as depression or anxiety, but concluded that there appeared to be evidence of corticocerebral dysfunctioning in anorexia nervosa. A recent study (Castro-Fornieles et al., 2009) comparing female adolescents showed differences in gray matter and cerebrospinal fluid but not in white matter volumes in the anorexic nervosa group. The increase in gray matter was related to a cortisol decrease, and the researchers concluded that these areas were affected more than white matter areas. They noted that nutritional recovery could reverse the gray matter changes. A longitudinal study of female adolescent anorexia nervosa (Stice & Bearman, 2001) has linked body image and eating-related risk factors that emerge during puberty to elevated rates of depression for adolescent girls. There are presently many studies investigating relationships between brain functioning and eating disorders, including ones that involve weight gain as well as loss.

Another severe condition that can become evident during this age period is adolescent-onset schizophrenia, in which the process of gray and white matter development is disrupted. Researchers have found that the rate of brain gray matter loss seems to be greater in certain brain areas such as the parietal, sensorimotor, and dorsolateral prefrontal cortices (Thompson et al., 2001). Douard and colleagues (2007) have reported that there may be both gray and white matter abnormalities in brain areas related to impairments in language and auditory perception. In contrast to earlier studies, they also found white matter alterations in primary motor cortex locations. They have interpreted these changes as indicating that there may be a loss of organization or alteration of myelin during adolescent brain development, and this may disrupt brain maturation and affect brain plasticity. More study of these developmental brain changes is needed, however, to understand this condition and to find ways to prevent such disruptions.

Suggestions for Fostering Brain Development and Learning

Adolescence is a time when many adults expect adult-like behaviors that are still only in the process of being fully developed. The articulateness and outwardly confident appearance of many adolescents may make such expectations seem appropriate. However, because of the continuing aspects of adolescent brain development, especially in areas of risk-taking, judgment, and social influence susceptibility, there is a continuing need for adults to monitor and support the brain development of adolescents.

For Families

- These years often present unique challenges for families as they deal with their adolescent's physical, mental, social, and behavioral changes. Because adolescents' brains are still reorganizing and restructuring, their skills may vacillate and, thus, many teen students may seem to be lazy, unmotivated, or conundrums. It is important to realize this and use that knowledge to determine whether to hold a teen accountable or just to accept that this is a feature of their stage in development.
- Teens engaging in risky behaviors that seem to be intensifying should be evaluated by appropriate personnel. If the risky behaviors could put the teen or others at risk, are found to be planned, take place on school property, or involve other students from school, school or city officials should be notified. Often, a referral to the school psychologist or school counselor may be helpful in figuring out how "normal" a teen's behavior is and what strategies can be recommended by that individual for use in the classroom and/or home.
- Because the changes to the structural organization of the brain cannot be physically viewed, parents may expect levels of competence or consistency from a teen that their brains cannot yet produce. More research is needed to understand functional implications of changes to their developing brains. Until then, parents should consider information on the adolescent's brain development stage when working with him or her.
- The impact of music, reading materials, movies, online media, video games, and television upon teen development has not been fully studied, but parents should review the types and quantity of their teen's media use.

For Educators

- Educators should provide supportive environments that help adolescents to advance their cognitive skills, leadership capabilities, and appropriate social behaviors. When designing teaching interventions, information about the adolescent brain and how it develops should be considered.

- If students seem to be exhibiting troubling behavior, discussing issues with parents and/or referring those students to school clinical personnel is essential so that intervention can take place in a timely manner. When parents are referred to a clinical professional, that individual should provide the parents with a clear idea of the approach that will be used, periodic progress reports, and an opportunity to decide whether the focus of the intervention needs to be heightened, changed, or stopped.

For Community Partners, Groups, and Policy Makers

- Most public policies include recognition of the fact that adolescents are not always fully aware of the consequences of their behaviors and thus, laws are usually written and judgments made that give adolescent offenders less severe or shorter consequences for risky behaviors that have resulted in harm to persons or property. However, there often is little follow-up or additional resources available to assist young offenders. Community groups and public agencies should accept child advocacy as part of their role in fostering the development of adolescents.
- Every community should have slightly risky but primarily safe venues in which adolescents can test their physical skills, cognitive abilities, and social relationships. For example, rock climbing walls, boating or ball playing areas, drama groups, photography clubs, socially secure areas, and other experiential venues allow adolescents to test their skills. Adult mentors who work with teens are valuable and should be available in all communities, not just in high-income suburban areas.

Case 3 Emma's Depression and Eating Disorder

In the past five years, the Kinley family has had their share of crises, including the death of Emma's beloved grandfather, her twin siblings' learning problems, and her dad's loss of employment, but they have come through them and seem to be in a more stable place. For example, her dad, a university professor, has found another teaching job; her mother, a pediatric nurse who works long hours, has searched for and found a care facility for her ailing mother, who survived the death of her husband; and Emma's twin brothers are getting extra services in school that are enabling them to do somewhat better. Emma's parents have often commented to others about how their achieving, stable, and low-maintenance daughter has been a joy throughout these years. Emma is a conscientious student, is involved in many school and extracurricular activities, holds a part-time job at a local store, and has a small group of close friends. She provides academic help for her brothers when they need it and often cooks dinner for the family in the evening. About four months ago, her mother noticed that Emily seemed to be getting thinner, and even though she made food for others in the family, her own portions were extremely small. She also restricted the types of food she would eat, usually just eating salads and other low-calorie food. However, since Emily seemed to be functioning well otherwise, her mother thought this was just a phase that would pass. As the months went by, Emily grew even thinner, spent most of her time in her own room, and cried often, even at very minor events going wrong. Her menstrual periods also disappeared. Finally, her parents took her to a counselor who diagnosed Emily's condition as depression and an eating disorder (anorexia nervosa) and made them aware of the seriousness of this condition. The counselor explained that these symptoms were often present in adolescence, especially in girls, and that they could become severe and lifelong problems if not treated early. Emily is now in group counseling and she has begun to try to eat more, although she is still not eating at normal levels. Her parents are wondering if their reliance on her to be the stable one in the family has had anything to do with her condition or whether it is a result of school or work pressures, some past experiences that she has yet to talk about, or problems with her friendship group at school. It seems strange to them that the child who seemed the most stable and strong has encountered this problem. She is continuing in counseling.

Case 4 Crystal's Executive Functioning

Crystal is one of those rare teenagers you meet who is a "bright light." She is full of stories, has positive energy, is smart and witty, and is always involved in events or projects at school. She plays soccer on a select team and was excited to start her first year of high school. Her teachers have found Crystal to have an endearing personality and a keen intellect as she added unique insights and contribution to class discussions. Crystal seemed to love the atmosphere, clubs, activities, and social environment. She did not have a boyfriend yet, but she and her friends talked about boys, and she thought she would have a boyfriend for the homecoming dance. She has seven class periods a day and also volunteers at an elementary school two times each week. Although her year started out well and she seemed to be flourishing socially and academically, her parents received a call from Mrs. Hanson, the English teacher, because Crystal was not getting assignments in on time and was behind on a major class project. The teacher learned that Crystal's parents also were having difficulty with their daughter and they felt her life now was "filled with chaos." Her mother confided that one day, Crystal broke down and said that she was struggling to keep her assignments in order, her locker clean, and her homework done. She stayed up late trying to get class reading done when, in the past, she had read easily. She complained that she could not keep everything straight in her head and she was having problems with friends who said that they were upset with her even though she didn't know why. Her dad said that the soccer coach had complained to him that Crystal wasn't concentrating on her game or remembering plays given to her and that she might not be a starter if she didn't improve. The teacher said that Crystal showed creative writing skills but had more difficulty completing reports that required planning and organization, and also that the social studies teacher noted that Crystal was having difficulty with organization and planning time. Mrs. Hanson assured the parents that other students starting high school sometimes experienced these problems and suggested they could help Crystal find support and direction. Crystal's parents agreed to meet with Mrs. Hanson and the school counselor to plan ways to help her gain better executive functioning skills.

Study Guide/Questions for Discussion

- Both Anita and Holden are having adjustment issues related to their high school experiences and, although these are relatively common problems, family members and educators might help them be more successful managing these issues during the high school years. Think about what strategies could help these students to have more enjoyable and productive experiences during adolescence and make suggestions for each of them.
- Both Emma and Crystal are facing greater difficulties during adolescence. Identify school and community resources that might help them and discuss how family, educators, and community members could provide effective resources and support for them as they face these issues.
- What aspects of the high school and community environments are most supportive of adolescent brain development and what aspects may be less

supportive? Give some suggestions of ways that the school environments and community resources could be more facilitative of optimum adolescent brain development.

Bibliography

Arain, M., Haque, M., Johal, L., Mathur, P., Nel, W., Rais, A., . . . Sharma, S. (2013). Maturation of the adolescent brain. *Neuropsychiatric Disease and Treatment, 9*, 449–461.

Baird, A. A., Gruber, S. A., Fein, D. A., MASS, L. C., Steingard, R. J., Renshaw, P. F., . . . Yurgelun-Todd, D. A. (1999). Functional magnetic resonance imaging of facial affect recognition in children and adolescents. *Journal of the American Academy of Child & Adolescent Psychiatry, 38*(2), 195–199.

Bava, S., & Tapert, S. F. (2010). Adolescent brain development and the risk for alcohol and other drug problems. *Neuropsychology Review, 20*(4), 398–413.

Blakemore, S. J., & Choudhury, S. (2006). Development of the adolescent brain: Implications for executive function and social cognition. *Journal of Child Psychology and Psychiatry, 47*(3–4), 296–312.

Bray, S., Krongold, M., Cooper, C., & Lebel, C. (2015). Synergistic effects of age on patterns of white and gray matter volume across childhood and adolescence. *eNeuro, 2*(4), 1–13.

Bronk, K. C. (2011). Neuropsychology of adolescent development (12 to 18 years old). In A. S. Davis (Ed.), *Handbook of pediatric neuropsychology* (pp. 47–57). New York: Springer.

Casey, B. J., & Jones, R. M. (2010). Neurobiology of the adolescent brain and behavior: Implications for substance use disorders. *Journal of the American Academy of Child & Adolescent Psychiatry, 49*(12), 1189–1201.

Castro-Fornieles, J., Bargalló, N., Lázaro, L., Andrés, S., Falcon, C., Plana, M. T., & Junqué, C. (2009). A cross-sectional and follow-up voxel-based morphometric MRI study in adolescent anorexia nervosa. *Journal of Psychiatric Research, 43*(3), 331–340.

Churchwell, J. C., & Yurgelun-Todd, D. A. (2013). Age-related changes in insula cortical thickness and impulsivity: Significance for emotional development and decision-making. *Developmental Cognitive Neuroscience, 6*, 80–86.

Compas, B. E., Orosan, P. G., & Grant, K. E. (1993). Adolescent stress and coping: Implications for psychopathology during adolescence. *Journal of Adolescence, 16*(3), 331.

Crews, F., He, J., & Hodge, C. (2007). Adolescent cortical development: A critical period of vulnerability for addiction. *Pharmacology Biochemistry and Behavior, 86*(2), 189–199.

Delvenne, V., Lotstra, F., Goldman, S., Biver, F., De Maertelaer, V., Appelboom-Fondu, J., . . . Mendelwicz, J. (1995). Brain hypometabolism of glucose in anorexia nervosa: A PET scan study. *Biological Psychiatry, 37*(3), 161–169.

Douard, G., Smith, S., Jenkins, M., Behrens, T. et al. (2007). Anatomically related grey and white matter abnormalities in adolescent-onset schizophrenia. *Brain, 130*, 2375–2386. doi:10.1093/brain/awm184.

Eshel, N., Nelson, E. E., Blair, R. J., Pine, D. S., & Ernst, M. (2007). Neural substrates of choice selection in adults and adolescents: Development of the ventrolateral prefrontal and anterior cingulate cortices. *Neuropsychologia, 45*(6), 1270–1279.

Giedd, J. N. (2008). The teen brain: Insights from neuroimaging. *Journal of Adolescent Health, 42*(4), 335–343.

Giedd, J. N., & Denker, A. H. (2015). The adolescent brain: Insights from neuroimaging. In J-P. Bourguignon et al. (Eds.), *Brain crosstalk in puberty and adolescence* (pp. 85–96). Switzerland: Springer International Publishing.

Giedd, J. N., & Rapoport, J. L. (2010). Structural MRI of pediatric brain development: What have we learned and where are we going? *Neuron, 67*(5), 728–734.

Gilmore, L., & Boulton-Lewis, G. (2009). 'Just try harder and you will shine': A study of 20 lazy children. *Australian Journal of Guidance and Counselling, 19*(2), 95–103.

Hall, G. S. (1904). *Adolescence* (2 vols). New York: Appleton.

Hines, A. R., & Paulson, S. E. (2006). Parents' and teachers' perceptions of adolescent storm and stress: Relations with parenting and teaching styles. *Adolescence, 41*(164), 597.

Khundrakpam, B. S., Lewis, J. D., Zhao, L., Chouinard-Decorte, F., & Evans, A. C. (2016). Brain connectivity in normally developing children and adolescents. *NeuroImage, 134*, 192–203.

Lerner, J. V., Phelps, E., Forman, Y. E., & Bowers, E. P. (2009). *Positive youth development*. Hoboken, NJ: John Wiley & Sons, Inc.

Levine, M. (2003). *The myth of laziness*. New York: Simon and Schuster.

Montemayor, R. (1983). Parents and adolescents in conflict: All families some of the time and some families most of the time. *Journal of Early Adolescence, 3*(1–2), 83–103.

Offer, D., Ostrov, E., Howard, K. I., & Atkinson, R. (1988). *The teenage world: Adolescents' self-image in ten countries*. New York: Plenum Medical Book.

Sebastian, C., Blakemore, S. J., & Charman, T. (2009). Reactions to ostracism in adolescents with autism spectrum conditions. *Journal of Autism and Developmental Disorders, 39*(8), 1122–1130.

Sebastian, C., Viding, E., Williams, K. D., & Blakemore, S. J. (2010). Social brain development and the affective consequences of ostracism in adolescence. *Brain and Cognition, 72*(1), 134–145.

Sherman, L. E., Payton, A. A., Hernandez, L. M., Greenfield, P. M., & Dapretto, M. (2016). The power of the like in adolescence: Effects of peer influence on neural and behavioral responses to social media. *Psychological Science, 27*(7), 1027–1035.

Sisk, C. L., & Foster, D. L. (2004). The neural basis of puberty and adolescence. *Nature Neuroscience*, 7(10), 1040–1047.

Sowell, E. R., Thompson, P. M., Holmes, C. J., Jernigan, T. L., & Toga, A. W. (1999). In vivo evidence for post-adolescent brain maturation in frontal and striatal regions. *Nature Neuroscience, 2*(10), 859–861.

Spear, L. P. (2000). The adolescent brain and age-related behavioral manifestations. *Neuroscience & Biobehavioral Reviews, 24*(4), 417–463.

Steinberg, L. (2005). Cognitive and affective development in adolescence. *Trends in Cognitive Sciences, 9*(2), 69–74.

Steinberg, L. (2010). Commentary: A behavioral scientist looks at the science of the adolescent brain. *Brain Cognition, 72*(1), 160–164. doi:10.1016/j.bandc.2009.11.003. NIH-PA.

Stice, E., & Bearman, S. K. (2001). Body-image and eating disturbances prospectively predict increases in depressive symptoms in adolescent girls: A growth curve analysis. *Developmental Psychology, 37*(5), 597.

Thompson, P. M., Vidal, C., Giedd, J. N., Gochman, P., Blumenthal, J., Nicolson, R., . . . Rapoprt, G. L. (2001). Mapping adolescent brain change reveals dynamic wave of accelerated gray matter loss in very early-onset schizophrenia. *Proc Natl Acad Sci USA, 98*, 11650–11655.

Urošević, S., Collins, P., Muetzel, R., Lim, K., & Luciana, M. (2012). Longitudinal changes in behavioral approach system sensitivity and brain structures involved in reward processing during adolescence. *Developmental Psychology, 48*(5), 1488.

Yurgelun-Todd, D. (2007). Emotional and cognitive changes during adolescence. *Current Opinion in Neurobiology, 17*(2), 251–257.

9

BRAIN DEVELOPMENT AND LEARNING IN THE ADULT YEARS

Case 1 John's Older Age Progress

Dr. John Black considered retiring from his position as a professor of mathematics when he reached the age of 65, but he decided that since he still loved his teaching role, was continuing to write and publish articles on mathematical issues, and had relatively good health, that he would continue working for a few more years. Thus, he remained in his university professor position until age 72 when his hearing (even with hearing aids) began to be a problem for understanding student comments in class. Because of his love for teaching, however, after his retirement he began to teach a course each semester for the older adult program that was sponsored by his university, drawing on his years of travel experience and interest in historical information to discuss the geography and history of various countries around the world and issues related to public affairs and policy. As he grew older, he found that his immediate memory for names of people and places began to fail and he began to have various other health problems (high blood pressure, osteoarthritis that made walking long distances and climbing stairs difficult), but his knowledge about mathematical, historical, and geographical information and his ability to convey such information while teaching was still excellent. He had a minor heart attack at age 80 but his recovery was excellent. At his present age of 87, he continues to be a great reader of current political information, to attend and comment on lectures, and to participate in a Facebook account. He still teaches an occasional class for the older adult program and he regularly attends his liberal church. He feels fortunate that his thinking power has enabled him to remain engaged and active even in his advanced years, particularly in the areas of knowledge in which he has always had great interest.

Case 2 Lela's Opioid Use and Its Effect on Her Children

Lela provides most of the care for her two children, Lloyd and Tina, because her husband, Jared, is a truck driver who travels extensively every week. He is usually home on weekends but sometimes not, depending on his travel assignments, and when he is home he often prefers relaxing by meeting some of his male buddies. The couple's children, Lloyd, age 5, and Tina, age 2, respectively, were developing well when Lela, age 35, was injured at her work as a health aide. She had to have major back surgery to remedy the injury. Lela's mother came in to help with the children during the period of the operation, but she could not stay long since she had other care responsibilities with her ill husband and younger son, who has major physical disabilities. Jared took off a few days from his work to care for Lela and the children, but he does not have extensive vacation time or leave time for family problems. During the weeks right after her operation, when Lela was in severe pain, she was given opioids by her doctor to help her cope with that pain. The healing process was lengthy and extensive, however, and Lela found that she really needed to have her pain prescription renewed regularly to feel well enough to take care of her many family and work responsibilities. Although Lloyd was in kindergarten and Tina was in daycare, both of those programs were half day, and thus, the children needed Lela's care the rest of the time. Unfortunately, Lela's opioid dependence began to interfere with her ability to show empathy and concern for her children's needs and to plan for their welfare. The kindergarten and the daycare teachers began to be concerned when the children came dressed inappropriately for the weather or when Lela did not make sure they were well fed or did not pick them up on time (daycare) or at the bus stop (kindergarten). Her doctor recently informed Lela that she could not have any more prescriptions for the opioid painkillers since they could cause long-term dependency, but Lela still feels that she needs help in coping with pain. At one of her work sites, she mentioned her concern about getting off the prescription opioids to a co-worker and that person said that he knew where she could get a cheap substitute that would work just as well. Lela is wondering if she should try this substitute to deal with her pain.

Review of Adult Brain Development

Contrary to earlier ideas about brain development, research now shows that there are many brain developmental processes still going on during the adult years. After studying the life course of adult brain development, Fjell et al. (2013) concluded "that most brain structures do not follow a simple path throughout adult life, and that accelerated decline in high age is not the norm of healthy brain aging" (p. 2). Some types of changes have been found to occur generally at various age levels, however. For example, during the young adult period (approximately age 21 to 39), the gray matter (GM) of the brain, which involves synaptogenesis, begins to decline, and this decline seems to be both constant and linear, while the white matter (WM) of the brain, which is involved in myelination, continues to increase in a quadratic pattern (e.g., doubled and maintained at that level) until about the age of 40, and then it begins to decrease quickly. Thus, although overall cerebral volume appears to be relatively stable during young adulthood, because of these two different trends, the apparent stability is due to the differing levels of activation in GM and WM during this age period. Also, the rates of GM and WM change seem to be relatively comparable between males and females (see Yulin et al., 2002 for further details).

In addition to studies comparing brain development in young adults and middle age adults, there also are some differences found in young adult brains as compared to adolescent brains. For example, adolescents may show less recruitment of the right ventral striatum (VS) and right-extended amygdala when anticipating gains in risky endeavors as compared with young adults (Bjork et al., 2004). That is, adolescents may be more likely than young adults to engage in risky behaviors and this may be due to adolescent delays in maturation of brain areas that assess risk, such as the ventral striatum, which is involved in affective processing and reward sensitivity (Qu et al., 2015). As these areas mature during young adulthood, risk-taking behaviors show declines. A recent study also has indicated a link between brain functioning related to smoking during adolescence and young adulthood. Musso and colleagues (2007) have reported that in young adults, the prefrontal attentional network activity was significantly reduced in smokers compared to nonsmokers, and the history of smoking duration (during adolescent and young adult years) was "directly related to the extent of diminished attentional network activity" (p. 159).

Recently there has been great interest in examining whether, where, and how neurogenesis may be occurring in the adult brain. At one time, it was assumed that all neurogenesis was completed by early adulthood. In 2002, after a review of studies of neurogenesis in birds and many other animals, Nottebohm stated, "It has been long assumed that the adult human brain is incapable of self-repair, yet there are no hard data that prove this point. It is possible that self-repair goes on in humans, but has gone undetected" (p. 746). Subsequent studies by other researchers are beginning to show that neurogenesis does occur during adulthood in certain parts of the brain, particularly in the dentate gyrus of the hippocampus (Jacobs, van Praag, & Gage, 2000). These authors found that when there are increased levels of serotonin, a neurotransmitter found primarily in the central nervous system and gastrointestinal tract, the rate of neurogenesis is enhanced; but when this process is disrupted by stress (and possible loss of sleep), it may contribute to clinical depression. Other researchers who also are studying synaptogenesis occurring in the adult brain are looking at how this process may contribute to the plasticity of the mature brain and assist individuals to adapt to changing environmental demands (Kelsch, Sim, & Lois, 2010). The possibility of neurogenesis contributing to plasticity of the brain at later age levels also has been noted by Aberg, Brywe, and Isgaard (2006), who assert that the growth hormone (GH)/insulin-like growth factor-I (IGF-I), secreted by somatotropic cells within the lateral wings of the anterior pituitary gland, may be involved in fostering neuroprotection and regeneration of neurons during adulthood.

According to Fjell et al. (2013), "the majority of brain structures follow complex, non-linear volumetric trajectories through adult life" (p. 9), and they advocate more longitudinal studies to gain understanding of these changes. Usually it is during the middle adult years (approximately age 40 to 55) when initial signs of brain developmental changes and possibly subsequent reductions in some types of abilities begin to be evident, although these changes may be very subtle. Different areas of the brain may show changes over middle and later adulthood, but there is a heterogeneous pattern. For example, Fjell and colleagues have indicated that the amygdala, putamen, thalamus, accumbens, and cerebellar cortex may show smaller linear reductions related to age, while the hippocampus, brain stem, and cerebellar WM may show accelerated decline from mid-life.

Research at later ages indicates that many brain-related changes occur in the age period between 50 to 65. For example, after age 60, total brain volume shows a decline (Fjell et al., 2013). Also, brain volume changes are greatly affected by medical conditions such as hypertension, cholesterol, diabetes, or other long-term problems related to genetics, and these conditions occur more often when adults are in this age range (see Scahill et al., 2003, for detailed information). By the old-age period (approximately 65 to 80), most researchers report significant changes in brain functioning, however. Since there also are a higher proportion of individuals living into their 90s or even 100s, study of brain functioning at these later ages is receiving greater and greater attention. Resnick and colleagues (2003) have indicated that although most older adults show brain tissue loss, there is "substantial variability" in its magnitude and they speculate that reduction in brain atrophy may be less in older adults who are medically and cognitively healthy. In one study comparing the source memory of older and younger adults, Cabeza and colleagues (2002) found that both young adults and those older adults who were low-performing on memory tasks used the right PFC brain regions, but older adults who were still high-performing engaged both the right and left PFC areas during the tasks. The researchers suggest that older adults may be able to continue higher memory performance by reorganizing their brain functions.

Impact of Genetic/Environmental Interactions During the Adult Years

As is the case at all ages, there are many genetic/environmental interactive factors that can affect brain development and functioning during the adult years. As noted earlier, many genetic factors may be present in younger adults that involve changes in brain functioning at later ages (Reiman et al., 2012). Some methods of improving or maintaining high brain functioning also have been identified. For example, recent research on the effects of vitamins have suggested that vitamin D (a neurosteroid) can positively influence various brain regulatory processes, even into older age levels (Kesby et al., 2011), and some researchers suggest that environmental influences such as extensive cognitive activity or specialized training can have a positive impact on brain structures and functions (Zatorre et al., 2012). In a study comparing the effects of education level and physical activity level, Ho and colleagues (2011) reported that there were 2–3% greater average tissue volumes in the temporal gray matter with each increment in educational level. That is, each additional amount of education the study participants had (some high school, high school, some college, college, and professional school) was related to their amount of brain gray matter. They also found that similar increases were found in the white matter of the corona radiata and parietal-occipital junction in relation to higher levels of physical activity. Thus, both mental and physical activity appeared to be related to higher levels of brain functioning. There also may be specific environmental enrichment activities, such as foreign language learning, that can contribute to healthier brain functioning. For example, Bialystok and colleagues (2004) have reported that controlled processing is carried out more effectively by bilinguals and that bilingualism helps to offset age-related losses in certain executive processes. They stated that "inhibitory processing, and working memory costs, reflecting the ability to deal with increasing task complexity, increased reliably with age, but these age-related increases were also reliably attenuated by bilingualism" (p. 299). Thus, bilingualism appears to influence not only language areas in the temporal lobe but also those in the frontal lobe.

The onset and severity of negative brain developmental changes may vary greatly among individuals, depending on both environmental and hereditary factors. Problematic conditions that are relatively common and may have genetic as well as environmental causes include schizophrenia in young adults, brain changes due to opioid use during young and middle adulthood, mid-adult frontotemporal dementia during middle adulthood, as well as Alzheimer's and other degenerative brain diseases occurring during later adulthood.

The diagnosis of schizophrenia often is made during the late adolescent or early adult time periods. However, Welham and colleagues (2008) have reported that many young adults who are eventually diagnosed with schizophrenia have shown symptoms of psychopathology during childhood and adolescence. They indicate that this "psychopathological trajectory" (p. 625) is correlated with a later diagnosis of schizophrenia. Seidman and colleagues (2006) have stated that, for persons with both genetic and environmental risk, investigation of the potential neuropsychological differences in family members with high risk should be undertaken during the adolescent age period. They state that there may be "critical neuromaturational changes during adolescence" (p. 511), and identification of these changes could give information and suggest strategies that might address the risk factors. They indicate that the young-adult age period (between 20 to 30) is the period of highest risk for this condition, although only about 5–10% of individuals at risk will develop schizophrenia. For those that do, however, the condition can be debilitating and affect their ability to work and engage in social relationships. For example, Angell and Test (2002) report that young adults who exhibit symptoms of this disease encounter difficulties in work environments and a loss of work-related and other supportive networks. This may result in dissatisfaction in social relationships and thus an increase in reported loneliness. Also, Agnew-Blais and Seidman (2013), in a meta-analysis of 30 studies, confirmed that "Neurocognitive dysfunction is a central feature of schizophrenia and is observed during all phases of the illness" (p. 1). Among the studies they reviewed, they reported that there were nine neurocognitive domains that showed at least some impairment, including general intelligence, attention, executive functioning, motor functioning, social cognition, visual-spatial ability, verbal/linguistic ability, memory, and cerebral asymmetry. They suggest that further study should investigate whether schizophrenia is due to a general cognitive deficit and that, because most of the research on this disorder suggests that early brain developmental and cognitive differences can be observed in individuals who show more extreme symptoms in young adulthood, attempts to ameliorate this disease should be addressed during childhood and adolescence.

Studies of opioid use have indicated that extended use may result in both current and long-term problematic effects on brain functioning. For example, Leppä and colleagues (2006) report that, when adults were given an opioid (remifentanil) in a research study, the brain regions that were most strongly activated included the rostral, mid-caudal, and caudal parts of the anterior cingulate cortex; the medial and inferior frontal gyri; and the precuneus. They note that these findings are similar to those of other PET studies of opioid effects, such as those of Petrovic et al. (2002) and Wagner et al. (2007). These studies reported that many areas of the brain (anterior cingulate cortex, prefrontal cortex, insula, and amygdala) are all involved in sensations related to pain and other distressful feelings. Leppa and colleagues noted that, in their studies, the major center activated by the opioid was in the posterior-superior part of the insular cortex. Because this area is involved in identifying the emotional significance of stimuli, evaluating distress, and regulating autonomic responses, as well as in evaluating ongoing experiences and emotions, they suggested that the effect of opioids on ability to understand one's own bodily reactions can be widespread and thus contribute to the dysfunctional behaviors often observed in persons with opioid addictions.

In an fMRI study on laser-evoked pain, Bingel and colleagues (2002) noted that activation was seen bilaterally in the amygdala. The amygdala, thalamus, and basal ganglia, including the caudate nucleus, are part of the opioid reward circuitry. Researchers have reported that the amygdala is activated by cocaine and nicotine as well as by other opioids (e.g., Breiter et al., 1997; Bingel et al., 2002). Langleben and colleagues (2015) indicated that heroin users showed reduced responsiveness in the amygdala, cuneus, caudate, and precentral gyrus and increased responsiveness in the medial frontal gyrus and precuneus. They conclude that opioid dependence may affect prefrontal and limbic cortical responses. Drug use also may be related to effects on parenting skills. Recently De La Cruz (2016) reported in an interview with researchers who have studied the effects of opioids that there may be an impairment of responsiveness to their children in parents with opioid dependence. For example, in one study, women on opioids did not produce expected responses to varied types of baby pictures (Langleben, 2015). That is, they were not able to "read" and respond to infant emotions portrayed in pictures.

According to Thies and Bleiler (2011), Alzheimer's disease (AD) now affects about 5.4 million people in the US, most of whom are over 65 years old. It is the most common form of dementia, and these authors predict that the number of cases will grow as more people live to advanced ages; thus, deaths related to AD are expected to increase. The most common initial symptom of AD is a gradual diminishment in ability to remember recently acquired information. In addition to memory problems, initial behavioral signs of AD include time and place confusion, misplacing items and not being able to find them, difficulty completing routine tasks, and problems in planning. As AD progresses, it may result in withdrawal from work or usual daily activities and changes in mood and personality. In its later stages, AD may result in disorientation, difficulty speaking or swallowing, problems in walking, and severely impaired judgment. Although other diseases such as Parkinson's may result in memory loss, initial symptoms of that disease are related to problems in movement rather than memory. The greatest risk factor for AD is advancing age, although this condition is not considered a normal stage in the aging process. Researchers are now suggesting that these AD symptoms may begin even 20 years earlier; however, not all people who have early symptoms progress to the later stages. There also may be familial, cognitive, cardiovascular, and head injury causal factors.

There have been many research studies of treatment effectiveness on these protein changes, but there has been no clear evidence that treating them improves the condition. In a review of such brain studies, Reitz (2012) indicates that while some study results support this hypothesis, there are also study results questioning these changes as causal. Recently, however, it has been reported (*60 Minutes*, CBS, Nov. 27, 2016) that a long-term double-blind study has been initiated to investigate whether past treatments have been started too late to be effective. This study has been initiated within a group of individuals in Columbia, many of whom carry a gene present in all Alzheimer's sufferers in this large family group. The study will investigate whether treatment initiated before the amyloid plaques are apparent in the brain can effectively prevent the disease. Some researchers have concluded that Alzheimer's disease may be the result of other neurodegenerative causes, however. For example, in a meta-analysis of genome-wide association studies, Lambert and colleagues (2013) have identified other "susceptibility loci" as possible triggers of this disease. Although there are no reliable treatments for AD, a number of drugs have been approved for improving symptoms, at least on a temporary basis. Healthy diets and continued social engagement are also recommended. Because of the extensive research being devoted to understanding and treating this disease, finding effective treatments or prevention methods has a high health-policy ranking, especially as the older adult population is increasing rapidly.

Frontotemporal dementia (FTD) is distinct from other dementias and Alzheimer's as it often strikes individuals who are not elderly but who are young adults, typically beginning in the mid-30s through 50 years of age. It only occurs in ten to fifteen out of 100,000 individuals (Coyle-Gilchrist et al., 2016). The changes that are first seen have less to do with memory and cognition than with often dramatic changes to their unique personality and behaviors. This type of dementia affects the frontal lobe of the brain, the area that is implicated in choice-making, attention, behaviors, and emotions. Recent research combined with neuroimaging correlates (Hutchings et al., 2017; Panchal et al., 2016) has shown that those with FTD have difficulty interpreting social rules, demonstrating socially appropriate behaviors, and losing social graces, manners, and emotional interpretations, including the ability to read the faces of others. There are various clinical subtypes that involve different symptoms (Mackenzie et al., 2010). Each involves different challenges, therapies, and management issues for those adults who have this condition.

Suggestions for Fostering Brain Development and Learning

Since brain development, both positive and negative, continues throughout life, the importance of continued attention to maintaining and enhancing healthy brains is now recognized. Families, educators, and community advocates can all support adult brain health.

For Families

- Families that encourage all members to continue to learn and have new experiences will be more likely to have healthy brain development, especially in the frontal lobe, during the adult years. Reading informational books, taking college courses or courses specifically designed for seniors, volunteering for activities in the community, and traveling abroad or within one's country to new places are ways to support the maintenance of a healthy brain.
- If family members observe an adult relative of any age exhibiting mental confusion or other symptoms that may be related to brain development problems, they should encourage that adult to have an assessment of the problems and follow treatment recommendations.
- Family members should not encourage overconsumption of alcohol or other legal drugs by family members and should not provide models of such overconsumption for younger family members. If a family member is having difficulty being a moderate user of such substances, the family should attempt intervention.

For Educators

- It is important for educators of young adults to realize that their brains are continuing to develop during these years, and thus provide challenging and stimulating environments that promote that development.
- As with families, educators who note that a young or older adult is having difficulty with cognitive understanding or memory should address these problems and potentially recommend assessment of the situation.

For Community Partners and Policy Makers

- Support for funding to study adult brain disorders should be ongoing and efforts to keep communities informed about such disorders and subsequent treatments should be supported.
- Treatment programs for adults with brain-related problems should be available in every community and for adults of all income levels.

Case 3 Adele's Puzzling Mental and Behavioral Problems

Adele is a 60-year-old retired executive who worked in the publishing industry, where she was known for her collaborative leadership style, quick wit and sarcasm, ease at social events, precise writing style, and unfailing attention to detail. In her spare time, she authored a column for the local newspaper, volunteered for local social charities, organized community events related to the arts, served on the voting board, read voraciously, drew with pencil and ink, and sent exquisite handwritten letters and cards to friends and family by mail. She planned to move to a retirement center in Arizona so that she would have new opportunities to explore and develop new friendships. However, shortly before moving, Adele began experiencing increasing difficulty with "word retrieval." This is the phenomenon that happens when an individual consistently has the feeling that they have a word on the "tip of their tongue" but cannot find and speak it when talking with others. Also, rather than continuing activities or finding new activities, Adele became indifferent and detached from what once had interested her. Her colleagues who were still in contact said it seemed Adele had become a totally different person. Her friends and family noticed that Adele began not only to forget words, but that she was gradually losing her capacity to carry on meaningful conversations and express ideas. Her difficulties gradually became worse in her new location. In fact, while she was initially an active participant in the resident council, Adele gradually stopped participating, and even stopped going to council meetings altogether. Along with her spoken-language issues, she became quieter and more socially reserved, and did not show much of the sarcastic quick wit she had been known for. When she did speak, it took Adele a long time to express herself and she occasionally made grammatical errors, something that had never happened before. Adele also started to have trouble writing but continued to doodle and draw. The problems she had with spoken and written language caused her a great deal of personal despair. Though her fellow residents were not intending to be harmful, it wasn't uncommon for others to remind her that she had trouble "spitting out her words." Even though Adele expressed profound disappointment regarding her speech and language, on the surface she maintained some of her social graces and seemed pleasant enough and "together" to many people. Although she recognized other people's faces, Adele developed the habit of looking downward rather than face-to-face. Because she was conscious of the changes she was experiencing, she developed major depressive symptoms. Over the next year, although she still participated in conversations, remembered long-term events, and doodled extensively, she talked in very short sentences, was emotionally aloof, and was very unsteady going down stairs. There was no history of dementia in her family and so this condition remained a mystery to them. However, her doctor labeled her condition "frontotemporal dementia."

Case 4 Isabel's Alzheimer's Progression

Isabel was age 67 when she began to have some concerns about her ability to remember the exact way to do financial and other routine procedures at the insurance office where she was an administrative assistant. To cope with these memory issues, she began writing down every type of procedure so that she would have a list to refer to when these memory lapses occurred, and that seemed to work pretty well for about a year. However, she also noted that the names of some of the clients were hard to remember, and her boss began to realize that she had forgotten to do a number of routine tasks and some clients' records were missing information. He met with her and stressed the importance of keeping good records, and he inquired about her health since she had always been such a careful worker. About that same time Isabel's husband, Doug, began to notice that she was showing lapses of memory and other problems of cognition at home, including forgetting to turn off the oven and stove burners, to call relatives when she had promised to do so, to take care of routine housekeeping activities, to take her medications, and to plan and carry through on social activities. He wondered if these symptoms were related to her previous diagnosis of diabetes. At the time of Isabel's 68th birthday, he suggested that it might be good for Isabel to discuss these memory and other problems with her doctor, Betty Baker. After the examination, Dr. Baker ordered a number of tests to investigate potential brain-related indicators of Isabel's cognitive difficulties. She reported that the results showed measurable changes in brain cerebrospinal fluid and some other symptoms that could indicate this condition was a mild early state of Alzheimer's disease (AD). Of course, this tentative diagnosis was very upsetting to Isabel and Doug because they both have had older relatives who progressed to more severe stages of AD. Dr. Baker indicated that she would continue to test biomarkers such as the level of beta-amyloid accumulation and the status of Isabel's brain nerve cells to determine whether and how quickly the disease was progressing, since progression differs in individuals. She also said that research is ongoing and there may be treatments found that will make progression of the disease less likely. Isabel is now 78, and over the past ten years her mental condition has deteriorated greatly. Her husband is now trying to come to terms with the possibility that Isabel's deteriorating cognitive and other disabilities due to this disease will require her to be placed in some type of care facility.

Study Guide/Questions for Discussion

- Find an article related to the role that advanced educational experiences and/or brain "games" may play in keeping the brain of older adults functioning well. Critique the article; that is, indicate which points or conclusions are based on sufficient research to make these valid and/or which assertions of the author may need to be further researched to be considered valid.
- Interview a social worker, psychologist, or other health professional who works with families in which a member is or has been an opioid user. Ask the professional's opinion about the conditions that promote such opioid use, how the use of opioids by adult family members may affect their children's positive developmental chances, what treatment methods are recommended, and which of these seem to be most effective.
- Review four journal articles discussing various types of adult dementia and the recent research on treatments and their results. Design a hypothetical study that could be done to gain more information about such conditions.

Bibliography

Aberg, N. D., Brywe, K. G., & Isgaard, J. (2006). Aspects of growth hormone and insulin-like growth factor-I related to neuroprotection, regeneration, and functional plasticity in the adult brain. *The Scientific World Journal, 6*, 53–80. doi:10.1100/tsw.2006.22.

Agnew-Blais, J., & Seidman, L. J. (2013). Neurocognition in youth and young adults under age 30 at familial risk for schizophrenia: a quantitative and qualitative review. *Cognitive neuropsychiatry, 18*(1-2), 44-82

Angell, B., & Test, M. A. (2002). The relationship of clinical factors and environmental opportunities to social functioning in young adults with schizophrenia. *Schizophrenia Bulletin, 28*, 259.

Bialystok, E., Craik, F. I., Klein, R., & Viswanathan, M. (2004). Bilingualism, aging, and cognitive control: Evidence from the Simon task. *Psychology and Aging, 19*(2), 290.

Bingel, U., Quante, M., Knab, R., Bromm, B., Weiller, C., & Büchel, C. (2002). Subcortical structures involved in pain processing: evidence from single-trial fMRI. *Pain, 99*(1), 313-321.

Bjork, J. M., Knutson, B., Fong, G. W., Caggiano, D. M., Bennett, S. M., & Hommer, D. W. (2004). Incentive-elicited brain activation in adolescents: Similarities and differences from young adults. *Journal of Neuroscience, 24*(8), 1793–1802.

Breiter, H. C., Gollub, R. L., Weisskoff, R. M., Kennedy, D. N., Makris, N., Berke, J. D. (1997). Acute effects of cocaine on human brain activity and emotion. *Neuron, 19*, 591-611.

Cabeza, R., Anderson, N. D., Locantore, J. K., & McIntosh, A. R. (2002). Aging gracefully: Compensatory brain activity in high-performing older adults. *Neuroimage, 17*(3), 1394–1402.

Coyle-Gilchrist, I. T., Dick, K. M., Patterson, K., Rodríquez, P.V., Wehmann, E., Wilcox, A., . . . Rowe, J. B. (2016). Prevalence, characteristics, and survival of frontotemporal lobar degeneration syndromes. *Neurology, 86*(18), 1736–1743.

Craik, F. I., Bialystok, E., & Freedman, M. (2010). Delaying the onset of Alzheimer disease Bilingualism as a form of cognitive reserve. *Neurology, 75*(19), 1726–1729.

De La Cruz, D. (2016, November 13). Opiods may interfere with parenting instincts, study finds. *New York Times*.

Fjell, A. M., Westlye, L. T., Grydeland, H., Amlien, I., Espeseth, T. et al. (2013). Critical ages in the life-course of the adult brain: Nonlinear subcortical aging. *Neurobiological Aging, 34*(10), 2239–2247. doi:10.1016/j.neurobiolaging.2013.04.006.

Ho, A. J., Raji, C. A., Becker, J. T., Lopez, O. L., Kuller, L. H., Hua, X., . . . & Thompson, P. M. (2011). The effects of physical activity, education, and body mass index on the aging brain. *Human Brain Mapping, 32*(9), 1371-1382.

Hutchings, R., Palermo, R., Piguet, O., & Kumfor, F. (2017). Disrupted face processing in frontotemporal dementia: A review of the clinical and neuroanatomical evidence. *Neuropsychology Review, 1*(27), 18–30.

Jacobs, B. L., van Praag, H., & Gage, F. H. (2000). Adult brain neurogenesis and psychiatry: A novel theory of depression. *Molecular Psychiatry, 5*(3), 262–270.

Kelsch, W., Sim, S., & Lois, C. (2010). Watching synaptogenesis in the adult brain. Annual *Review of Neuroscience, 33*, 131–149. doi:10.1146/annurev-neuro-060909-153252.

Kesby, J. P., Eyles, D. W., Burne, T., & McGrath, J. T. (2011). The effect of Vitamin D on brain development and adult brain function. *Molecular and Cellular Endocrinology, 347*(1–2), 121–127. doi:10.1016/j.mce.2011.05.014.

Lambert, J. C., Ibrahim-Verbaas, C. A., Harold, D., Naj, A. C., Sims, R., Bellenguez, C., . . . Grenier-Boley, B. (2013). Meta-analysis of 74,046 individuals identifies 11 new susceptibility loci for Alzheimer's disease. *Nature Genetics, 45*(12), 1452–1458.

Langleben, D. D. (2015). Buprenorphine-naloxone treatment of prescription opioid abuse: Does past performance predict future results? *The Journal of Clinical Psychiatry, 76*(2), 195–197.

Leppä, M., Korvenoja, A., Carlson, S., Timonen, P., Martinkauppi, S., Ahonen, J., . . . Kalso, E. (2006). Acute opioid effects on human brain as revealed by functional magnetic resonance imaging. *Neuroimage, 31*(2), 661–669.

Mackenzie, I. R., Neumann, M., Bigio, E. H., Cairns, N. J., Alafuzoff, I., Kril, J., & Ince, P. G. (2010). Nomenclature and nosology for neuropathologic subtypes of frontotemporal lobar degeneration: An update. *Acta neuropathologica, 119*(1), 1.

Musso, F., Bettermann, F., Vucurevic, G., Stoeter, P., Konrad, A., & Winterer, G. (2007). Smoking impacts on prefrontal attentional network function in young adult brains. *Psychopharmacology, 191*(1), 159–169.

Nottebohm, F. (2002). Neural replacement in adult brain. *Brain Research Bulletin, 57*(6), 737–749.

Panchal, H., Paholpak, P., Lee, G., Carr, A., Barsuglia, J. P., Mather, M., . . . Mendez, M. F. (2016). Neuropsychological and neuroanatomical correlates of the Social Norms

Questionnaire in frontotemporal dementia versus Alzheimer's disease. *American Journal of Alzheimer's Disease & Other Dementias®*, *31*(4), 326–332.

Petrovic, P., Kalso, E., Petersson, K. M., & Ingvar, M. (2002). Placebo and opioid analgesia-imaging a shared neuronal network. *Science, 295*(5560), 1737-1740.

Qu, Y., Galvan, A., Fuligni, A. J., Lieberman, M. D., & Telzer, E. H. (2015). Longitudinal changes in prefrontal cortex activation underlie declines in adolescent risk taking. *The Journal of Neuroscience, 35*(32), 11308–11314.

Reiman, E. M., Quiroz, Y. T., Fleisher, A. S., Chen, K., Velez-Pardo, C., Jimenez-Del-Rio, M., . . . Giraldo, M. (2012). Brain imaging and fluid biomarker analysis in young adults at genetic risk for autosomal dominant Alzheimer's disease in the presenilin 1 E280A kindred: A case-control study. *The Lancet Neurology, 11*(12), 1048–1056.

Reitz, C. (2012). Alzheimer's disease and the amyloid cascade hypothesis: a critical review. *International Journal of Alzheimer's Disease*, 2012.

Resnick, S. M., Pham, D. L., Kraut, M. A., Zonderman, A. B., & Davatzikos, C. (2003). Longitudinal magnetic resonance imaging studies of older adults: A shrinking brain. *Journal of Neuroscience, 23*(8), 3295–3301.

Scahill, R. I., Frost, C., Jenkins, R., Whitwell, J. L., Rossor, M. N., & Fox, N. C. (2003). A longitudinal study of brain volume changes in normal aging using serial registered magnetic resonance imaging. *Archives of Neurology, 60*(7), 989–994.

Seidman, L. J., Thermenos, H. W., Poldrack, R. A., Peace, N. K., Koch, J. K., Faraone, S.V., & Tsuang, M. T. (2006). Altered brain activation in dorsolateral prefrontal cortex in adolescents and young adults at genetic risk for schizophrenia: an fMRI study of working memory. *Schizophrenia Research, 85*(1), 58-72.

Thies, W., & Bleiler, L., & Alzheimer's Association Report. (2011). Alzheimer's disease facts and figures. *Alzheimers Dement*, 7(2), 208–244.

Wagner, K. J., Sprenger, T., Kochs, E. F., Tölle, T. R., Valet, M., & Willoch, F. (2007). Imaging Human Cerebral Pain Modulation by Dose-dependent Opioid AnalgesiaA Positron Emission Tomography Activation Study Using Remifentanil. *The Journal of the American Society of Anesthesiologists, 106*(3), 548-556.

Welham, J., Isohanni, M., Jones, P., & McGrath, J. (2008). The antecedents of schizophrenia: a review of birth cohort studies. *Schizophrenia Bulletin, 35*(3), 603-623.

Yulin, G., Grossman, R. L., Babb, J. S., Rabin, M. L., Mannon, L. J., & Kolson, D. L. (2002). Age-related total gray matter and white matter changes in normal adult brain. Pt. I: Volumetric MR imaging analysis. *American Journal of Neuroradiology, 23*, 1327–1333.

Zatorre, R. J., Fields, R. D., & Johansen-Berg, H. (2012). Plasticity in gray and white: neuroimaging changes in brain structure during learning. *Nature Neuroscience, 15*(4), 528

10

USING NEUROIMAGING AND NEURODIAGNOSTIC TECHNIQUES TO UNDERSTAND AND IMPROVE BRAIN FUNCTIONING

Case 1 Roger's School Phobia

Roger was the Lytle family's second child and very different from his outgoing older sibling, Logan. Even as an infant he had a strong startle reflex and was easily upset by loud noises. However, his parents accommodated their child-rearing style to his temperament, giving him advanced warnings of routine changes and confidence-building activities. When he was 6 years old, his parents moved to a new house but they kept his old routines and familiar toys. Although new experiences made him anxious, he did not show severe symptoms during first and second grade. When Roger's brother transitioned to middle school, however, and Roger had to go on the bus to third grade without Logan, he began to resist going to school each morning. He would say he was feeling sick, but when his mother let him stay home, his sick feelings disappeared. He said mean kids were on the bus so she drove him to school, but then had trouble getting him out of the car. She had to deposit him forcefully at the school as he screamed and begged not to go in. She thought that there must be trouble with other children or teachers, so she discussed Roger's anxiety with his teacher and principal and they investigated but could not find any clear reason for Roger's anxiety. They said, however, that he did not have friends to sit with at lunch and his school performance was being affected by anxiety. His parents asked Roger about school experiences and to tell them what was making him feel anxious, but he was not able to express reasons. Because Roger's severe and persistent anxiety-related and avoidance behavior was interfering with his functioning, his parents contacted a neuropsychologist. The specialist gave Roger some assessment tests and suggested that there might be hyperactivity in the amygdala area of Roger's brain. His parents are considering whether to have him take a neuroimaging test that the specialist recommended. A cognitive behavior plan was designed for Roger, which enabled him to begin to face his anxiety and, with special school accommodations, be able to participate in most third-grade activities. However, he has many mornings when his anxiety is extremely high and he resists attending school, especially on testing days.

Understanding the Brain's Metabolic and Magnetic Activity

Neuroimaging refers to an increasing number of methods that produce images of the interactions among structures, functions, and communication systems of the brain. Although structures of the brain have been well defined, many brain functions are not yet well understood and exact locations of brain areas involved in specific functions are only beginning to be clarified. Neuroimaging methods are used increasingly by physicians and neuropsychologists to investigate brain functioning in persons with brain deterioration diseases, such as Alzheimer's; to discover neural circuitry underlying behavioral patterns of children with neurodevelopmental disorders; to learn brain functioning effects of accidents, such as TBI; and to investigate possible disease conditions, such as strokes and brain tumors. Other neuropsychological theorists are learning more about typical cognitive processes, using these techniques to investigate structure/function interactions in normal brain development. There have been many advancements in neuroimaging procedures, and the information they provide is beginning to be helpful to investigate effects of various diseases on brain structures and to understand the role of brain interactivity during common socioemotional and cognitive processes.

At present, however, the use and effectiveness of these techniques are still being evaluated and considered experimental (e.g., PET). Investigators recently have revealed common mistakes, errors, and limitations of statistical methods and software associated with neuroimaging (e.g., An et al., 2015; Hupe, 2015). Wintermark and colleagues (2013) note that use of imaging techniques assessing brain tissue effects of strokes must be evaluated for congruence with the stroke focus area and cost of the procedure. They state that much research data on neuroimaging of brain conditions is drawn from group comparisons using data collected from typical subjects, and this evidence is not sufficient for clinical use with individual patients. Poldrack (2006) has cautioned cognitive researchers that presently, the only appropriate inferences to be drawn from neuroimaging study data are those involved in examining which brain areas are activated during the engagement of certain cognitive processes. He advises that the practice of "reverse inference," in which researchers conclude that when a certain part of the brain has been activated, this means an identifiable cognitive process is occurring, is not appropriate. Although these types of inferences may be eventually confirmed, Poldrack notes that they go beyond what current neuroimaging procedures can achieve. A review of neuroimaging techniques shows both achievements and potentials of these methods.

Neuroimaging and Neurodiagnostic Techniques

Positron Emission Tomography (PET)

This procedure focuses on identifying brain metabolic receptors associated with specific neurotransmitters. Chemicals are injected into the bloodstream and then the participant performs short, nonactive tasks while measures are taken of blood flow, oxygen, and glucose metabolism in the working brain. It is often used to diagnose tumors, the early onset of Alzheimer's disease, and learning problems such as ADHD (del Campo et al., 2013). The procedure localizes brain activity at the centimeter range and thus is not as precise as some other methods. It can be used on young children but does expose them to radioactive materials.

Single-Photon Emission Computerized Tomography (SPECT)

This procedure is similar to PET but involves the use of Gamma rays emitting radioisotopes to measure cerebral blood flow. It often is used to diagnose epilepsy and other conditions involving seizures, as well as traumatic brain injuries (Henderson & Morries, 2014). As with PET, it is noninvasive and can be used on young children; however, it exposes participants to radioactive materials.

Magnetic Resonance Imaging (MRI)

This procedure uses the resonance of sound images from magnetic fields and radio waves to investigate blood flow. It is often substituted for X-rays. The machine is noisy and participants must lie very still within a cramped environment, so it requires orientation to the equipment, especially for children and older individuals. Some participants find it difficult to endure, and researchers have made attempts to make it easier by providing movies or other media to watch during the procedure. It does not expose participants to radiation. It has been used often in studies investigating typical brain development of newborns, toddlers, and preschoolers (Almi, 2015) and of elementary age children through adolescence (Durston et al., 2001), as well as for investigating conditions such as ADHD (Mahone et al., 2011).

Functional Magnetic Resonance Imaging (fMRI)

This procedure involves using the paramagnetic properties of oxygenated hemoglobin, and it provides images of changing blood flow in the brain during neural activity and post processing of the data through statistical programming to obtain an enhanced and colorful image. Participants do mental tasks that can reveal perceptions and actions within the brain. It has similar conditions of noise and participant stillness in a cramped environment, as MRI does, but it can localize areas of the brain in millimeters so it is helpful in diagnosis. It has also been used in studies of cognitive and brain maturational changes during late childhood and adolescence (Luna et al., 2001). Figure 10.1 shows a child's fMRI results.

Diffusion Tensor Imaging

Diffusion tensor imaging (DTI) is an advanced application of magnetic resonance imaging (MRI) that is especially sensitive to injuries in the microstructure of

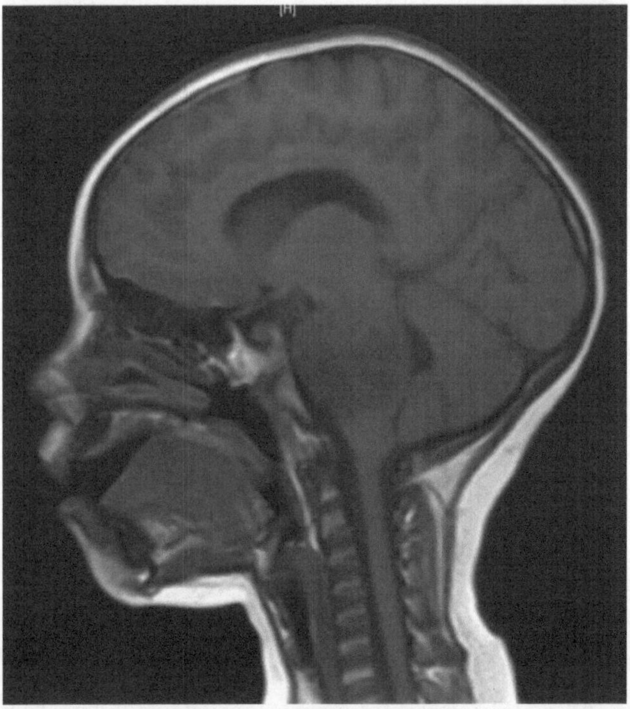

FIGURE 10.1 Pediatric MRI Showing a Brain Stem Tumor

white brain matter. It measures intensity, direction, and movement of water molecules. However, even slight movement of participants can cause distortion, and images may be blurry due to low spatial resolution. It is used to investigate concussions and the extent of diffuse axonal injury, and to predict recovery time; and it has been applied to studying unique brain circuitry associated with cognitions and behaviors related to neurodevelopmental disorders such as autism (Hazlett et al., 2017), dyslexia (Koerte et al., 2016), and pediatric TBI (Roberts et al., 2016). Figure 10.2 shows an adult's DTI results.

Magnetic Source Imaging/Magnetoencephalography (MSI/MEG)

In this procedure, the magnetic field products of the electrical activity of the brain are directly observed. To image even weak neuromagnetic signals successfully, it involves magnetically shielded rooms and advanced techniques for signal processing. Because the procedure reads signals near the brain surface, deeper brain issues cannot be studied. However, it gives good spatial and temporal data in surface

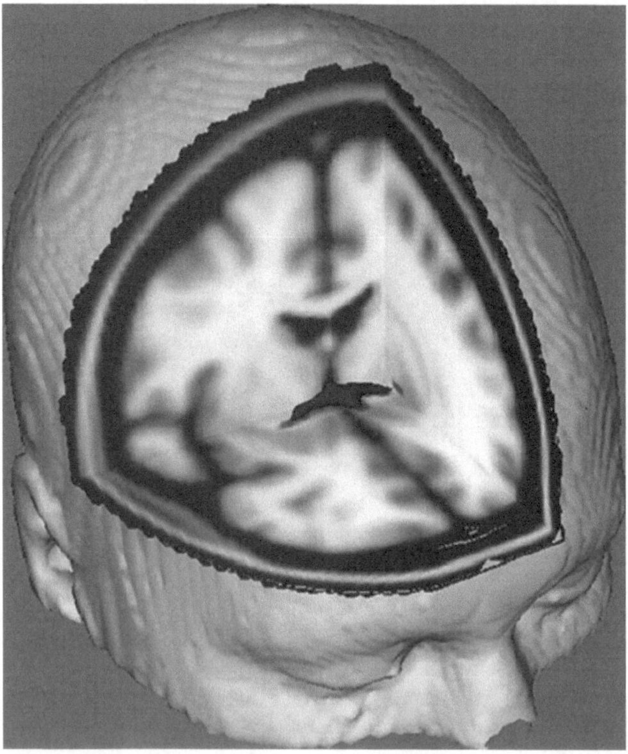

FIGURE 10.2 Adult DTI Showing the Anterior Commissure Within the Brain

areas with less distortion, yielding information about spatial-temporal rhythms or patterns in populations having reading, spoken language, seizures, and attention problems (Dimitriadis et al., 2016; Wehner, 2007).

Other Neuroimaging Procedures

Other procedures for specific brain investigations include diffuse optical imaging (DOI), which uses infrared light to generate images and measures optical absorption of hemoglobin due to variations in oxygen levels; event-related optical signal (EROS) also uses infrared light to observe optic fibers. Cranial ultrasound is used in neonate brain investigations since, at that period of life, the brain has open fontanelles. It does not use radiation so it is a safer procedure for neonates. There is also a new procedure involving cerebral organoids, which are referred to as "mini-brains" (Dias & Guillemot, 2017), and this procedure may provide clues about the neurogenesis of brain development, especially in the forebrain regions. To construct these brain structures, clusters of stem cells are manipulated "to self-organize through endogenous patterning events that mimic the developing brain *in vivo*" (Renner et al., 2017, p. 7). This technique may use a noninvasive source, such as skin cells from an individual with a neurodevelopmental disorder, to see how external and internal factors influence the mini-brain's structure and how it differs from typical brain development.

Psychologically-Based Neurodiagnostic Techniques

Before the use of neuroimaging techniques became prevalent, localization of brain injuries and lesions relied upon EEG's, X-rays, neuropsychological exams, and neuropsychological experts' interpretation of major ways of diagnosing focal areas of brain dysfunction (Ruff, 2003). In the late 1800s, physicians such as Broca (1865) and Wernicke (1874) established direct brain-behavior relationships involving production of speech and comprehension of language. They then associated premorbid behavioral changes in patients with focal infarcts revealed during post-mortem studies. About 70 to 80 years ago, the use of psychometric assessments of specific brain-behavior relationships began, resulting in the "Period of Neuropsychological Localization" (Ruff, 2003, p. 848). Application of neuropsychological methods drew upon results of invasive research with animal subjects that established specific brain-behavior connections. If a certain brain area was involved in a type of animal behavior (e.g., aversion to food, aggression toward siblings), neuropsychologists would assess their patient using standardized techniques, and then use inferences made from testing results to interpret their patient's behavior as having its origin in a brain area that had been reported to be involved in a section of the research animal's brain.

As computerized topography became available in the 1970s, the use of neurodiagnostic techniques to localize brain damage lessened. Because diagnostic tests and methods often measure more than one type of behavior, and because many behaviors involve concerted activity in a range of brain areas, these methods were less able to isolate specific brain areas that might be affected. Instead, the focus of the neuropsychologist turned from attempting to localize behavior to using neurodiagnostic instruments to infer brain-behavior relationships across human domains of performance. Today, when data are collected on an individual, the current clinician is better positioned to interpret and "map" neuropsychological functioning, make recommendations for targeted interventions, and improve that individual's cognitive health. Psychological and neuropsychological instruments can be divided by their category of human functioning, as indicated by the eight domains in the acronym "*ICE SEALS*." They include **I**ntellectual/**C**ognitive, **E**xpressed Verbal and Language, **S**patial and Visual, **S**ensorimotor, **E**xecutive Functioning, **A**ttention and Working Memory, **L**earning and Memory, and **S**ocial-Emotional and Behavioral. Representative tests or instruments from each domain are shown in Table 10.1.

TABLE 10.1 Neurodiagnostic Instruments

Intellectual/Cognitive
Universal Nonverbal Intelligence Test (UNIT)
Differential Ability Scales, Second Edition (DAS-II)
Stanford-Binet Test of Intelligence—Fifth Edition (SB-V)
Bayley Scales of Infant Intelligence, Third Edition (Bayley-III)
Wechsler Intelligence Scale for Children—Fifth Edition (WISC-V)
Reynolds Intellectual Assessment Scales—Second Edition (RIAS-II)
Kaufman Assessment Battery for Children, Second Edition (KABC-II)
Wechsler Preschool and Primary Scales of Intelligence—Fourth Edition (WPPSI-IV)
Woodcock-Johnson Tests of Cognitive Ability—Fourth Edition (WJ-IV, Cognitive)
Expressed Verbal and Language Skills
Preschool Language Scale, Fourth Edition (PLS-IV)
Comprehensive Test of Phonological Processing (CTOPP)
Test of Language Competence—Extended Version (TLC-E)
Clinical Evaluation of Language Function, Fourth Edition (CELF-IV)
Kaufman Test of Educational Achievement, Second Edition (KTEA-II)
Developmental Neuropsychological Instrument (NEPSY-II), Selected Subtests
Woodcock-Johnson Tests of Oral Language—Fourth Edition (WJ-IV, Oral Language)
Selected Subtests from the WISC-V, WJ-IV, DAS-II, SB-V, and other instruments
Spatial and Visual
Judgment of Line Orientation (JLO)
Developmental Neuropsychological Instrument (NEPSY-II), Selected Subtests
Selected Subtests from the WISC-V, WJ-IV, DAS-II, SB-V, and other instruments
Sensorimotor
Dynamometer
Fingertip Tapping Test
Purdue Pegboard Test (PPT)
Grooved Pegboard Test (GPT)

Tactual Performance Test (TPT)
Dean-Woodcock Sensory-Motor Battery (DWSMB)
Wide Range Assessment of Visual-Motor Abilities (WRAVMA)
Developmental Visual Motor Integration, Fifth Edition (DVMI-V)
Selected Subtests from the WISC-V, DAS-II, NEPSY-II, and other instruments

Executive Functioning
Trail-Making Test (TMT)
Rey Complex Figure Test
Tasks of Executive Control (TEC)
Wisconsin Card Sorting Test (WCST)
Stroop Color-and-Word Test (STROOP)
Delis-Kaplan Executive Functioning System (D-KEFS)
Behavioral Rating Inventory of Executive Functioning Scales (BRIEF)
Developmental Neuropsychological Instrument (NEPSY-II), Selected Subtests

Attention
Trail-Making Test (TMT)
Test of Everyday Attention, Child Version (TEA-Ch)
Continuous Performance Test—Second Edition (CPT-II)
Conners Continuous Performance Test, Second Edition (CCPT-II)
Selected Subtests from the WISC-V, DAS-II, NEPSY-II, and other instruments)

Learning and Memory
Children's Memory Scales (CMS)
Test of Memory and Learning, Second Edition (TOMAL-2)
California Verbal Learning Test, Children's Version (CVLT-C)
Developmental Neuropsychological Instrument (NEPSY-II), Selected Subtests
Wide Range Assessment of Memory and Learning, Second Edition (WRAML-2)
Selected Subtests from the WISC-V, WJ-IV, DAS-II, SB-V, and other instruments

Presently, neurodiagnostic techniques include both behavioral tests and neuroimaging methods. Professionals in neuropsychological fields provide interpretation of neurodiagnostic techniques and recommend diagnostic instruments that enable them to diagnose brain difficulties. Guidelines for such tests are described in Chapter 12. As noted by Tonkonogy and Puente (2009), "Historically, neuropsychological studies existed without reference to brain- imaging studies and vice versa. Over the last decade the two have interfaced, resulting in exciting discoveries and a greater understanding of brain dysfunction" (p. 20).

Application of Neuroimaging and Neurodiagnostic Research

Neuroimaging techniques are used extensively to help researchers and practitioners learn more about typical and atypical brain functioning, and these methods are gaining increasing importance. As Poldrack (2006) has noted, however, the techniques are not yet appropriate for accurately identifying certain areas of the brain responsible for specific cognitive processes—both because such processes are complex and may involve many areas of the brain, and because the techniques are still relatively imprecise. Although these techniques hold promise for diagnosing and predicting how brain areas may be affected by disease or injury, at present the application of research to practice is still in early stages. Results are useful in conjunction with neuropsychological evaluations to give diagnosticians additional insight into the prognosis and treatment of many diseases that affect brain functioning. Research studies investigate both which areas of the brain are activated when certain types of experiences are presented, and developmental differences in brain structures and functions at various age levels. Also, studies are investigating brain activation differences in individuals with learning problems, diseases involving brain functioning, and other conditions. Some findings have been discussed in earlier chapters. This chapter includes additional examples.

Neuroimaging Research on Typical Brain Functioning

An increasing number of neuroimaging studies focus on examining areas of the typical brain activated by emotional and cognitive stimuli of various types. Zeki and Romaya (2008), for example, have focused on brain areas activated by emotions. In one of their studies they reported that when adults were shown pictures that usually elicit feelings of hate, the right putamen, premotor cortex, medial insula, and fronto-medial gyrus showed activity. They contrasted this to studies of areas of the brain activated when feelings of love and caring were elicited, and indicate that the brain areas activated during feelings of hate were primarily different from those activated by positive emotions, although the putamen and insula were activated in both conditions. In another of their studies of brain activation during emotional experiences, they reported that for couples in loving relationships, the same brain areas were activated by both partners (Zeki & Romaya, 2010).

Various types of cognitive functioning have been studied by neuroimaging techniques. Eichenbaum and Cohen (2004) investigated brain areas activated in declarative memory and reported that the hippocampus was involved in rapid encoding of associations between stimulus events and contexts, encoding these as sequences of events, and linking them to networks that support inferential memories. Smith and Jonides (1999) discussed sites involved in executive functioning, especially those that involve memory processes, and they noted that storage of verbal materials activates Broca's area and other left-hemisphere and premotor areas, while storage of spatial information activates the right-hemisphere premotor cortex; object information activates other areas of the prefrontal cortex; and selective attention and task management activate the anterior cingulate and dorsolateral prefrontal cortex. Owen and colleagues (2005) also have investigated working memory and report consistent activation of frontal and parietal cortical regions. Bush, Luu, and Posner (2000) note that both cognitive and emotional processing involve the anterior cingulate cortex (ACC), and they describe how it plays a part in a circuit involving attention and regulation of both cognitive and emotional processing. Other recent neuroimaging studies also discuss complex links between cognitive and emotional processing. In a study of specific cognitive processes involved in word reading, Fiez and Petersen (1998) reported that left-lateralized regions in occipital and occipito-temporal cortex, the left frontal operculum, bilateral regions within the cerebellum, primary motor cortex, superior and middle temporal cortex, and medial regions in the supplementary motor area and anterior cingulate all showed activation. Evidence from these studies is a reminder that the brain operates as a whole, even though certain areas may be primary activation sites.

Numerous neuroimaging studies of specific brain areas related to various diseases or other debilitating conditions also have been reported. There are numerous studies on the effects of TBI (traumatic brain injury) and Alzheimer's disease on brain structures and functions. Belanger and colleagues (2007) investigated whether neuroimaging methods such as fMRI, PET, and SPECT are more effective than MRI and CT scans when examining effects of mild TBI, and suggest these newer methods may provide better information. Azouvi (2000) also has noted that such methods are more effective in relating cognitive and behavioral evidence of traumatic brain injury to the prefrontal-cingulate network of the brain. Zhang and colleagues (2012) reviewed the use of neuroimaging techniques with Alzheimer's patients and report that they enable examination of brain area effects, such as senile plaques, neurofibrillary tangles, cortical atrophy, neuronal loss, and vascular damage, as well as changes in brain biochemistry. Bakker and colleagues (2007) have discussed gait disorders in Parkinson's disease and indicate that the basal ganglia-thalamo-cortical system appears to be related to this problem. They indicate that there are problems using PET, fMRI, and EEG with Parkinson's patients because these techniques require subjects to stop movement during the tasks related to cerebral activity and suggest using MEG and transcranial magnetic stimulation (TMS), which provide direct measures of neural activity. Neuroimaging techniques are often used in conjunction with neuropsychological treatments. For example, Holzschneider and Mulert (2011), in a review of neuroimaging studies related to anxiety, discussed how these can be used in relation to treatments such as exposure-based therapy and pharmacological treatment options.

Another area in which neuroimaging studies have been helpful is in charting development change in the brain from prenatal to older-adult age periods. Findings from many of these studies have been reported in other chapters, but some information is briefly reviewed here.

Developmental Findings

Researchers have used neuroimaging studies to observe the nature of brain development and brain functioning during various age periods. Almli and colleagues (2007) studied the normal brain development of infants and toddlers using MRI techniques, and Luna and colleagues (2001) have used fMRI studies to investigate brain development from childhood to adolescence. Their studies show increased activation in the frontal, parietal, striatal, and thalamic areas of the brain as age increases. They note that the prefrontal area is more active in adolescents than in children, and the lateral cerebellum is more active in adults than in adolescents. Thus, they conclude that brain maturation trends are evidence of cognitive development throughout these age periods. Neuroimaging studies such as these are now beginning to contribute much to understanding of brain development and the meaning of changes at various ages.

Infant and Toddler

Neuroimaging plays a role in evaluating brain development of infants, especially premature infants. El Dib and colleagues (2010) reported that abnormality in both white matter and gray matter gyral maturation can be observed in MRIs of premature infants. Hintz and O'Shea (2008) indicate there are still controversies over whether early evaluations using neuroimaging techniques should be routinely used, however. Using fMRI methods, Dehaene-Lambertz and colleagues (2006) studied how 3-month-old infants begin to acquire their native language. They studied the brain regions that were active during normal and reversed speech in awake and sleeping infants. They found that left-lateralized brain regions (e.g., superior temporal and angular gyri) that are similarly activated for language in adults were already active in infants. Awake infants who heard speech also had activation in the right prefrontal cortex. The researchers concluded that the "precursors of adult cortical language are already active in infants, well before the onset of speech production" (p. 2013).

Preschool

According to Brown and Jernigan (2012), there have not been many neuroimaging studies focused on preschool children because it is difficult to do such studies with "young, unsedated children" (p. 1). Thus, although infant studies are common, preschool studies are less available, leaving "a substantial gap in the evidence for the preschool period" (p. 1). The types of studies that have been reported with preschoolers typically investigate potential brain development problems, such as attention deficit (Mahone et al., 2011) or autism (Wolff & Piven, 2013). These studies show some atypical early brain development in such children. Mahone and colleagues found that reduced left caudate volume and anomalous basal ganglia play a role in early-onset symptoms of ADHD, and Wolffe and Piven note that increased gray and white matter and amygdala volumes, as well as some aberrant connectivity factors, may show a disrupted brain development pattern in children who develop autistic symptoms. This research is at a very early level, however, so it is not yet definitive.

Elementary Age

Some fMRI studies comparing elementary age children and adults give insights into how areas of the brain develop over that time. Booth and colleagues (2001) looked at differences in brain activation during tests of orthographic and phonologic representations and found developmental differences between adults and 9- to 12-year-old children as they made judgments about spelling and rhyming tasks. Although they report that both groups showed activation in the left inferior frontal gyrus during the tasks, adults had greater activation in that area, indicating that there are developmental increases in the magnitude of activation during development. Using fMRI technology, Wu and colleagues (2013) looked at potential sex and intelligence differences in brain network maps of elementary age children and found age-related increases in frontal brain regions and decreases in the parietal, temporal, and occipital brain regions. They noted that boys had "significant higher values of the global efficiency" (p. 1) but there were no significant IQ-related differences. Positive correlations between IQ and regional nodal properties were found in the attention system and negative correlations were found in brain regions related to emotion and language. Although most findings related to elementary age children's brain development are preliminary, this study did focus on how the functional brain networks of healthy children are developing.

Middle Childhood

During this age period, there are still major developmental changes in brain structure and functioning. According to Klingberg, Forssberg, and Westerberg (2002), fMRI studies indicate that there is an increase in working memory during middle childhood. They studied children and adolescents between the ages of 9 and 18 as they performed visuospatial and baseline tasks and found that the superior frontal and intraparietal cortex in the older children were more activated. Frontal and parietal areas are involved in controlling attention and spatial working memory. Development of these functions over the middle childhood period plays an important role in mature cognitive development. Reactions of children of this age to painful and non-painful visual stimuli also have been investigated, and researchers found that perception of others' pain increased hemodynamic activity in the neural circuits that process first-hand individual pain experiences (e.g., insula, somatosensory cortex, anterior midcingulate cortex) but also in brain areas related to social and moral behavior (e.g., temporo-parietal junction, amygdala). Although these results are similar to adult results, the researchers suggest further study is needed with children who exhibit social cognitive disorders because they often seem deficient in experiencing empathy and guilt (Decety et al., 2008).

Adolescence

There are also changes in the brain during adolescence that are being understood with neuroimaging techniques. Giedd (2008) reports that longitudinal neuroimaging studies show that during adolescence, there are declines in brain gray matter as well as increases in both functional and structural connectivity. In the adolescent brain, there is a change in the balance between frontal lobe and limbic/subcortical functions, and this process continues into young adulthood. Presently the influence of marijuana use by adolescence has been of interest to researchers since that use is relatively widespread. Schweinsburg and colleagues (2010) found in an fMRI study that on memory tasks, recent users showed greater response in the medial and left superior prefrontal cortices, as well as in the bilateral insula. They concluded that marijuana use disrupts neural connections associated with spatial working memory and thus results in compensatory brain responses. However, marijuana users who had abstained for a short time period before the test showed responses similar to nonmarijuana users. Long-term effects were not studied.

Adulthood

Neuroimaging studies have also found developmental change in brain maturational structures into young adulthood. Lebel and Beaulieu (2011) used diffusion tensor magnetic resonance imaging in a study with participants aged 5 to 30 to note axonal packing and myelination over that time. They reported that the frontotemporal connections developed more slowly into adulthood. They did not find statistically significant gender differences. Many cognitive tasks become more difficult at older ages and Cabeza and colleagues (2002) were interested in what compensatory mechanisms older adults might use to keep their memories functioning. They investigated this question using PET scans of younger and older participants in a set of memory tasks, comparing PFC activity in younger adults with PFC activity of two types of older adults: ones with memory problems and ones who showed no memory problems, to see if they accessed different areas of the brain in performing recall and source memory tasks. They found that while both young adults and older adults with memory problems accessed the right PFC, high-performing older adults used both PFC areas bilaterally. They concluded that there was evidence of "plastic reorganization of neurocognitive networks" (p. 1,394) in the older adults who still had good memory functioning.

Suggestions for Fostering Brain Development and Learning

For Families

- Since there is still much to be learned about brain development, families who are willing to let their typically developing children participate in neuroimaging research studies focused on brain development issues can assist researchers in understanding brain development. Thus, they can play a role in helping increase knowledge of brain development.
- If their child exhibits severe emotional, social, or cognitive difficulties, families should seek assistance from neuropsychologists who can assess those difficulties

and determine what interventions might be helpful for the child. They should seek help early rather than waiting until problems are greater because intervention may be most effective during the early years of brain plasticity.

For Educators

- Educators should inform themselves about various assessment and intervention techniques that can help children with learning problems or other developmental issues evident in school. They should not base their assessments on popular information about "left/right brains" or any other pseudoscientific information.
- It is important for educators to work collaboratively with school psychologists, speech pathologists, and other specialists in their system and to initiate the practices they recommend for children who have brain-related learning needs in their classrooms.

For Community Partners, Groups, and Policy Makers

- Funding support for neuroimaging studies related to both typical development and treatment of brain-related illnesses should be a priority for these groups. As more information is discovered, the brain health of the society will be strengthened.
- Policy makers should use evidence from brain research when devising strategies to improve the brain health of individuals in the society.

Study Guide/Questions for Discussion

- Interview a school psychologist, speech pathologist, or other professional who uses information from neuroimaging studies. Ask them about what is helpful presently and what would be useful new research that would assist them in fostering healthy brain development.
- Select a developmental age (e.g., infant, adolescent) and read five published neuroimaging studies about that age level. Write a brief report outlining findings about brain development from these studies and discuss implications of that information for practice.

Bibliography

An, H. J., Seo, S., Kang, H., Choi, H., Cheon, G. J., Lee, D. S., . . . Lee, J. S. (2015). Quantitative evaluation of improved MR-based attenuation correction for brain PET/MRI studies. *Journal of Nuclear Medicine, 56*(Suppl 3), 95.

Alami, B. (2015, January). Magnetic resonance imaging findings and Spectrum of Etiologies in children epilepsy. European Congress of Radiology 2015.

Almli, C. R., Rivkin, M. J., McKinstry, R. C., & Brain Development Cooperative Group. (2007). The NIH MRI study of normal brain development (Objective-2): Newborns, infants, toddlers, and preschoolers. *Neuroimage, 35*(1), 308–325.

Azouvi, P. (2000). Neuroimaging correlates of cognitive and functional outcome after traumatic brain injury. *Current Opinion in Neurology, 13*(6), 665–669.

Bakker, M., Verstappen, C. C. P., Bloem, B. R., & Toni, I. (2007). Recent advances in functional neuroimaging of gait. *Journal of Neural Transmission, 114*(10), 1323–1331.

Belanger, H. G., Vanderploeg, R. D., Curtiss, G., & Warden, D. L. (2007). Recent neuroimaging techniques in mild traumatic brain injury. *The Journal of Neuropsychiatry and Clinical Neurosciences, 19*(1), 5–20.

Booth, J. R., Burman, D. D., Santen, F. W.V., Harasaki, Y., Gitelman, D. R., Parrish, T. B., & Mesulam, M. M. (2001). The development of specialized brain systems in reading and oral-language. *Child Neuropsychology*, 7(3), 119–141.

Broca, P. (1865). *Sur le siège de la faculté du langage articulé* (Vol. 6, pp. 337–393). Paris: V. Masson.

Brown, T. T., & Jernigan, T. L. (2012). Brain development during the preschool years. *Neuropsychology Review, 22*(4), 313–333.

Bush, G., Luu, P., & Posner, M. I. (2000). Cognitive and emotional influences in anterior cingulate cortex. *Trends in Cognitive Sciences, 4*(6), 215–222.

Cabeza, R., Anderson, N. D., Locantore, J. K., & McIntosh, A. R. (2002). Aging gracefully: Compensatory brain activity in high-performing older adults. *Neuroimage, 17*(3), 1394–1402.

Decety, J., Michalska, K. J., & Akitsuki, Y. (2008). Who caused the pain? An fMRI investigation of empathy and intentionality in children. *Neuropsychologia, 46*(11), 2607–2614.

Dehaene-Lambertz, G., Hertz-Pannier, L., & Dubois, J. (2006). Nature and nurture in language acquisition: Anatomical and functional brain-imaging studies in infants. *Trends in Neurosciences, 29*(7), 367–373.

del Campo, N., Fryer, T. D., Hong, Y. T., Smith, R., Brichard, L., Acosta-Cabronero, J., . . . Dowson, J. (2013). A positron emission tomography study of nigro-striatal dopaminergic mechanisms underlying attention: Implications for ADHD and its treatment. *Brain, 136*(11), 3252–3270.

Dias, C., & Guillemot, F. (2017). Revealing the inner workings of organoids. *The EMBO Journal, 36*(10), 1299–1301, e201796860.

Dimitriadis, S. I., Laskaris, N. A., Simos, P. G., Fletcher, J. M., & Papanicolaou, A. C. (2016). Greater repertoire and temporal variability of Cross-Frequency Coupling (CFC) modes in resting-state neuromagnetic recordings among children with reading difficulties. *Frontiers in Human Neuroscience*, 10.

Durston, S., Pol, H. E. H., Casey, B. J., Giedd, J. N., Buitelaar, J. K., & Van Engeland, H. (2001). Anatomical MRI of the developing human brain: What have we learned? *Journal of the American Academy of Child & Adolescent Psychiatry, 40*(9), 1012–1020.

Eichenbaum, H., & Cohen, N. J. (2004). *From conditioning to conscious recollection: Memory systems of the brain* (No. 35). Oxford: Oxford University Press on Demand.

El-Dib, M., Massaro, A. N., Bulas, D., & Aly, H. (2010). Neuroimaging and neurodevelopmental outcome of premature infants. *American Journal of Perinatology, 27*(10), 803–818.

Fiez, J. A., & Petersen, S. E. (1998). Neuroimaging studies of word reading. *Proceedings of the National Academy of Sciences, 95*(3), 914–921.

Giedd, J. N. (2008). The teen brain: Insights from neuroimaging. *Journal of Adolescent Health, 42*(4), 335–343.

Hazlett, H. C., Gu, H., Munsell, B. C., Kim, S. H., Styner, M., Wolff, J. J., Elison, J. T, Swanson, M. R., Hongtu, Z., Botteron, K. N., Collins, D. L., Constantino, J. N., Dager, S. R., Estes, A. M., Evans, A. C., Fonov, V. S., Gerig, G., Kostopoulos, P., McKinstry, R. C., Pandey, J., Paterson, S., Pruett, J. R., Jr., Schultz, R. T., Shaw, D. W., & Zwaigenbaum, L. (2017). Early brain development in infants at high risk for autism spectrum disorder. *Nature, 542*(7641), 348-351

Henderson, T. A., & Morries, L. D. (2014). SPECT perfusion imaging demonstrates improvement of traumatic brain injury with transcranial near-infrared laser phototherapy. *Advances in Mind-Body Medicine, 29*(4), 27–33.

Hintz, S. R., & O'Shea, M. (2008, February). Neuroimaging and neurodevelopmental outcomes in preterm infants. *Seminars in Perinatology, 32*(1), 11–19.

Holzschneider, K., & Mulert, C. (2011). Neuroimaging in anxiety disorders. *Dialogues in Clinical Neuroscience, 13*(4), 453–461.

Hupé, J. M. (2015). Statistical inferences under the Null hypothesis: Common mistakes and pitfalls in neuroimaging studies. *Frontiers in Neuroscience, 9*(18), 1–9.

Klingberg, T., Forssberg, H., & Westerberg, H. (2002). Increased brain activity in frontal and parietal cortex underlies the development of visuospatial working memory capacity during childhood. *Journal of Cognitive Neuroscience, 14*(1), 1–10.

Koerte, I. K., Willems, A., Muehlmann, M., Moll, K., Cornell, S., Pixner, S., . . . Shenton, M. E. (2016). Mathematical abilities in dyslexic children: A diffusion tensor imaging study. *Brain Imaging and Behavior, 10*(3), 781–791.

Lebel, C., & Beaulieu, C. (2011). Longitudinal development of human brain wiring continues from childhood into adulthood. *Journal of Neuroscience, 31*(30), 10937–10947.

Luna, B., Thulborn, K. R., Munoz, D. P., Merriam, E. P., Garver, K. E., Minshew, N. J., . . . Sweeney, J. A. (2001). Maturation of widely distributed brain function subserves cognitive development. *Neuroimage, 13*(5), 786–793.

Mahone, E. M., Crocetti, D., Ranta, M. E., Gaddis, A., Cataldo, M., Slifer, K. J., . . . Mostofsky, S. H. (2011). A preliminary neuroimaging study of preschool children with ADHD. *The Clinical Neuropsychologist, 25*(6), 1009–1028.

Owen, A. M., McMillan, K. M., Laird, A. R., & Bullmore, E. (2005). N-back working memory paradigm: A meta-analysis of normative functional neuroimaging studies. *Human Brain Mapping, 25*(1), 46–59.

Poldrack, R. A. (2006). Can cognitive processes be inferred from neuroimaging data? *Trends in Cognitive Sciences, 10*(2), 59–63.

Renner, M., Lancaster, M. A., Bian, S., Choi, H., Ku, T., Peer, A., . . . Knoblich, J. A. (2017). Self-organized developmental patterning and differentiation in cerebral organoids. *The EMBO Journal*, e201694700.

Roberts, R. M., Mathias, J. L., & Rose, S. E. (2016). Relationship between diffusion tensor imaging (DTI) findings and cognition following pediatric TBI: A meta-analytic review. *Developmental Neuropsychology, 41*(3), 176–200.

Ruff, R. M. (2003). A friendly critique of neuropsychology: Facing the challenges of our future. *Archives of Clinical Neuropsychology, 18*(8), 847–864.

Schweinsburg, A. D., Schweinsburg, B. C., Medina, K. L., McQueeny, T., Brown, S. A., & Tapert, S. F. (2010). The influence of recency of use on fMRI response during spatial working memory in adolescent marijuana users. *Journal of Psychoactive Drugs, 42*(3), 401–412.

Smith, E. E., & Jonides, J. (1999). Storage and executive processes in the frontal lobes. *Science, 283*(5408), 1657–1661.

Tonkonogy, J. M., & Puente, A. E. (2009). *Localization of clinical syndromes in neuropsychology and neuroscience*. New York: Springer Publishing Company.

Wehner, D. T., Ahlfors, S. P., & Mody, M. (2007). The influence of semantic processing on phonological decisions in children and adults: A Magnetoencephalography (MEG) study. *Journal of Speech, Language, and Hearing Research, 50*(3), 716–731.

Wernicke, C. (1874). *Der aphasische Symptomencomplex: eine psychologische Studie auf anatomischer Basis*. Breslau: Cohn.

Wintermark, M., Sanelli, P. C., Albers, G. W., Bello, J., Derdeyn, C., Hetts, S. W., . . . Rowley, H. (2013). Imaging recommendations for acute stroke and transient ischemic attack patients: A joint statement by the American Society of Neuroradiology, the American College of Radiology, and the Society of NeuroInterventional Surgery. *American Journal of Neuroradiology, 34*(11), E117–E127.

Wolff, J. J., & Piven, J. (2013). On the emergence of autism: Neuroimaging findings from birth to preschool. *Neuropsychiatry, 3*(2), 209–222.

Wu, K., Taki, Y., Sato, K., Hashizume, H., Sassa, Y., Takeuchi, H., . . . Kawashima, R. (2013). Topological organization of functional brain networks in healthy children: Differences in relation to age, sex, and intelligence. *PloS One, 8*(2), e55347.

Zeki, S., & Romaya, J. P. (2008). Neural correlates of hate. *PloS One, 3*(10), e3556.

Zeki, S., & Romaya, J. P. (2010). The brain reaction to viewing faces of opposite-and same-sex romantic partners. *PloS One, 5*(12), e15802.

Zhang, L., Chang, R. C., Chu, L. W., & Mak, H. K. (2012). Current neuroimaging techniques in Alzheimer's disease and applications in animal models. *American Journal of Nuclear Medicine and Molecular Imaging, 2*(3), 386–404.

11

USING EEG AND ERP METHODOLOGY TO UNDERSTAND AND IMPROVE BRAIN FUNCTIONING

Case 1 Erich's Puzzles and Video Game Play

Ever since Erich was a little boy, he has loved solving puzzles. He started with wooden puzzles with the pegs, but quickly moved into 24-piece and then 48-piece puzzles. Noticing how adept he was at putting together puzzles, his parents began mixing two and three puzzles together for him to figure out. He also was quick to pick up Lego building skills. Sometimes his parents would just watch him, but many times they would talk with him during his play, intuitively using prepositional terms like "next to, on, beside, and through." At older ages, Erich showed a love for video games. He could do many moves and achieve goals in the games that his parents couldn't achieve. In school, it was no surprise that Erich achieved extremely high scores in math. His standardized test scores were always at the top of the scale and his teachers had to think of new and creative ways of challenging him. For half the year during his second and third grade years, Erich attended the third and fourth grade classrooms for math class. Even with this enrichment, Erich still seems bored in class, but he continues to demonstrate his unique mathematical abilities. Erich's parents received a flyer for a video game study in which Erich would play a video game while wearing a net on his head. For participating in the study, he would receive a gift card to his favorite pizzeria. Since Erich loved to play video games, this seemed like a great opportunity for him to learn a little about scientific research and do something he liked. So, his parents signed him up. At the lab, Erich was fitted for the correct size net and given directions on how to play the video game, which was a simplified Tetris game where he was shown different-shaped pieces in different rotational patterns in space and asked whether the piece fit in a specific space. Before playing the game, he was given a math test, shown his brain wave patterns, and asked questions about how computers worked and how his brain worked. After 15–20 minutes of playing the video game, Erich completed another math test, and then was given his gift card and thanked for his time. The researchers who worked with Erich noticed how well he had done on the math portion of the experiment and decided to compare Erich's ERP results to the rest of the group's ERP results to find out if there was a difference in areas of cortex activation, latency of wave component onset, wave amplitude, or wave frequency in Erich's brain in comparison to results in these brain areas of other children in the study. They compared the information from this study to information from other spatial-reasoning-oriented video games to learn whether some types of video games are more proficient at increasing spatial reasoning abilities in young children.

Understanding the Brain's Electrical Activity

Electroencephalography or EEG is a measure of electrical activity on the scalp, which is distinguished from single-cell unit recordings where electrodes are placed on particular cells in the brain (in facial recognition, for example; Quiroga et al., 2014). Electrical activity received by the electrodes at the scalp passes through brain tissue and is deflected at multiple angles when it reaches the skull. Thus, it is difficult for EEG researchers to say for certain exactly where the source of the electrical activity comes from, which is one of the major disadvantages of this technique. However, current researchers have increased the number of electrodes used, increasing the spatial resolution in high-density recording methods. When 128 electrodes or more are used, researchers can statistically identify source generators in the brain, thus making it possible to localize the source of electrical activity. Figure 11.1 shows electrode placement for ERP studies.

One way to examine EEG data is through wavelet analysis. In this type of analysis, the electrical waves are measured as the number of wave phase cycles per second, or Hertz (Hz). There are five well-researched EEG bands: Delta, 0–4Hz; Theta, 4–8Hz; Alpha, 8–12Hz; Beta, 12–30Hz; Gamma, 30–150Hz. Recent research has split several of these into upper and lower bands based on their

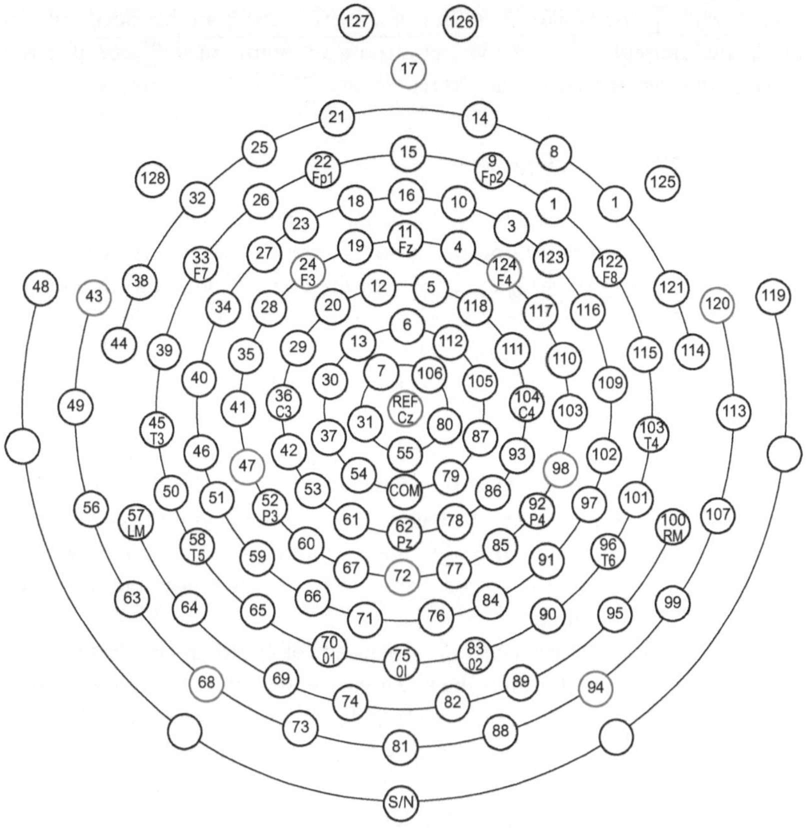

FIGURE 11.1 EGI 128 Channel Sensor Net Layout Version 1.0

respective theorized cognitive function. These bands were named for their respective Greek letters in the order in which they were discovered, meaning Alpha waves have been examined for the longest time. As neuroscience research progressed, each of the bandwidths became associated with specific cognitive processes. Delta waves are primarily seen during the first two years of life, while Theta waves occur prominently during sleep (Pizzagalli, 2007). Alpha waves, which are corollaries of Mu waves (sensorimotor rhythms), show increases from childhood to adolescence and are often apparent in the posterior brain regions (occipital and parietal lobe areas) during resting times or during alertness. Gamma waves, which are studied specifically on their sub-band, are relatively short bursts typically associated with the firing of single neurons during the active mode of a neural circuit (Buzsáki & Wang, 2012). While there is ongoing debate as to the function of these waves, two uses of monitoring Gamma EEG are clear. First, detection of these waves in certain areas can help in the identification of certain brain diseases (Sanei & Chalmers, 2007). Second, coordination of Gamma with other wave frequencies like Theta in other areas of the brain has been linked to coordinated muscular activity and seems to be an important indicator of sensory and cognitive events (Basar et al., 2001).

EEG and ERP Techniques

Almost 90 years ago, a scientist by the name of Hans Berger developed several experiments in which he demonstrated how to measure the electrical activity of the brain. Recording of electrical activity of the brain through the placement of small electrodes on the scalp produces an electroencephalogram (EEG) that can be interpreted to understand brain activity. Such electrophysiological recordings have been popular in brain research because these techniques are relatively noninvasive and inexpensive, and the method is regarded by many scientists as the most efficient way of measuring developmental changes due to its functional use from birth to late adulthood. A typical procedure for using the EEG technique is to record EEG during specific events designed to measure cognitive processing and then make comparisons with the EEG recorded during rest periods or when no environmental stimulation is offered. EEG can be recorded over a relatively long time, from seconds to minutes.

When the goal is to produce a brief snapshot of electrical brain activity for a discrete stimulus or set of stimuli, the researcher will use the ERP, or event-related potential technique. ERPs are the preferred method of uncovering the neural basis for language problems associated with developmental dyslexia (Lyytinen et al., 2005) and have been used extensively in evaluating reading (Jang, Kang, & Kim, 2015), language proficiency (Andersson et al., 2014), linguistics (Pélissier, Krzonowski, & Ferragne, 2015), and executive functioning (Espinet, Anderson, & Zelazo, 2012). ERPs are time-locked, which means that researchers can mark and measure the onset of the particular waves of interest and then look at statistical analysis, usually through analysis of variance (ANOVA) and regression techniques. ERPs are the averaged time-locked wave responses embedded within the EEG signal.

ERP researchers collect many samples of brain activity when a participant is doing a designated task and then examine that average (the ERP). The procedure is similar to having a child take a ten-question math test 50 times and averaging the results for answers to the ten questions over the 50 attempts. That average would more likely provide a solid picture of the child's math performance on those ten questions. Similarly, but because there are statistical imperfections in the ERP technique, many trials (usually more than 100) are needed to eliminate the background EEG electrical activity. After that is eliminated, only segments with specific responses to the particular stimulus (i.e., related to the question being studied) are observable (Bell & Cuevas, 2012). Then researchers can evaluate hypotheses, make predictions, and potentially create theory as to what cognitive processes are occurring in the brain when certain stimuli are presented.

Application of ERP Research

An ERP experiment usually is analyzed in several ways. Most developmental ERP studies have focused on the typical oddball paradigm with an infant habituation paradigm (DeBoer, Scott, & Nelson, 2007). Another typical ERP experiment gaining traction is the Go/NoGo task. In this experiment, participants respond by clicking a button when they see a specific stimulus, like an X presented in 70% of the trials, and do not respond when they see another stimulus, like an O presented in 30% of the trials. Because ERPs are time-locked, the sine waves presented are the average of all participants on every trial for each of the two situations. The sine waves are labeled for positive or negative amplitude and at the time (in milliseconds) from stimulus onset. For example, the P100 or P1 is the first positive amplitude peaked wave occurring after time 0. N2 is named as it would be the second negative amplitude average waveform occurring 200 ms after the stimulus onset. Its amplitude has been linked to response inhibition. In the NoGo of one Go/NoGo example, the N2 amplitude decreases with age in the frontal and central areas of the brain.

While researchers are interested in the peak amplitudes of waves, they are also concerned with several other measurable aspects of ERPs. In fact, deflections in the ERP (referred to as components) reflect specific aspects of sensory and cognitive processes associated with various stimuli (DeBoer, Scott, & Nelson, 2007). Cognitive neuroscientists can look for similarities or differences between experimental conditions. The wave's onset is referred to as its latency, which can also be measured and compared. In one example, Johnstone and colleagues (2006) found that there was a significant developmental difference in the peak latency of the P300, or P3, ERP waveform in the parietal lobe (Pz) in the NoGo situation. As this difference was correlated with reaction time and accuracy on the Go task, they theorized that the P3 latency is related to efficient Go and NoGo processing. They stated that while younger children seem to demonstrate greater mental efforts, older children may have more efficient neural activation processes than younger children, at least in this task.

Other measurable aspects of EEG/ERP data are joint time frequency (JTF), wavelet analysis, and source localization techniques. An analysis using JTF is typically based on a variation of the Fourier Transform, which commonly plots the magnitude or phase content of a signal as a function of frequency. Thus, the Fourier Transform allows examination of the frequency-domain view of a signal. This transformation provides information about a signal that might not be immediately apparent from an examination of the signal in its raw time-domain representation. Examining EEG data in the frequency domain is very useful in gaining a better understanding of the electrical signal. As work by Mulert et al. (2010) demonstrates, for example, wave amplitudes can be deconstructed through the joint time-frequency spectrogram, giving a clearer illustration of the frequency of the wave components that make up the amplitude of the signal. This analysis provides a more in-depth statistical and visual microscope into examining the cooperation between specialized and widely distributed areas that are a prerequisite of higher cognitive functions and large-scale neuronal integration (Herrmann, Grigutsch, & Busch, 2005). Wavelet analysis replaces action potentials, measured in microvolts (μV), for wave frequency (Hz) on the y axis keeping time (ms) as the x axis.

Developmental Findings

This methodology also has contributed much to understanding of brain development and the meaning of changes at various ages. Some of these studies have been reported in earlier chapters and others are discussed here.

Infants and Toddlers

The use of EEG is widely viewed as the best neuroimaging technique for developmental studies because it is noninvasive, resistant to motor artifacts, and can be applied to sensitive populations such as newborns (Taylor & Baldeweg, 2002; see also Winkler et al., 2008). While EEG research is typically performed in a clinical setting focusing on diagnosis and treatment of neurological diseases like epilepsy, EEG can also be used to assess brain impairments and cognitive functions (de Haan, 2007), creating a link between behavioral and brain development. Usually, newborn waking EEG hovers in the Delta and Theta bands while Alpha and Beta increase with developmental maturity well into adolescence and adulthood, respectively.

The Mu rhythm is the 8–12Hz frequency band exhibited over the sensorimotor cortex (scalp positions C3 and C4, for example). The rhythm is attenuated during periods of goal-directed action or observation of goal-directed actions (Pineda, 2005). Mu in the sensorimotor cortex, or inferior parietal, is associated with motor control and movement mirror neurons. Cuevas and colleagues (2014) reviewed findings and methodological considerations for research in infant Mu rhythm EEG and noted that there is greater Mu activation among infants who have had experience performing an action when they later observe or perform the same action. This effect is attenuated when children observe videos of the action. That is, infants are cognitively less engaged when watching a video of an action than when the action is performed by a live person (van Elk et al., 2008). This suggests that infant actions are processed semantically and these semantic representations are incorporated into the mirror neuron system, which is mediated by social context and social cues (Choisdealbha & Reid, 2014). These researchers suggest that the mirror neuron (motor) system coordinates with systematic functions of the verbal or semantic meaning-making system, which makes the words adults speak to infants equally as important as the visual model they provide. An interdisciplinary group of developmental neuroscientists (Filippi et al., 2016) found that Mu desynchronization during action execution predicted infants' later propensity to reproduce experimenter's goal-directed behavior. They state that this provides the first evidence that motor system activation predicts imitation of other individuals' goals during infancy.

Most ERP research with infants has focused on cognitive developmental issues (Nelson & Monk, 2001; Blair, Zelazo, & Greenberg, 2005), linguistic development (see Molfese & Molfese, 2000), and more recently on the influence of infant stress (for a review, see Ursache & Noble, 2016). ERP research also has focused on language processing in children with autism who show language delays. Kuhl et al. (2005) investigated language development of children with autism spectrum disorder (ASD) compared to a typically developing control group of children in the age range of 32 to 53 months (M = 45.3). Using an auditory preference test that had "motherese" and non-speech similar-speech sounds, they tested for phonetic discrimination with mismatch negativity (MMN). Children with ASD who demonstrated preference for the non-speech condition did not show a significant MMN when syllables changed, while children who preferred the motherese showed MMN reactions similar to controls. This research supports other recent findings that demonstrate a difference linguistic processing and social processing in infants with ASD.

Preschool

The 3 to 5 age period is enormously important for cognitive growth and synaptic pruning. Neuroimaging studies have focused on cognitive processing in children. Liu and colleagues (2009) report that the development of theory of mind by children also coincides with a linear change in the brain where specialization occurs as the brain matures. In a foundational longitudinal study of children aged 6 months to 16 years, Brown and Jernigan (2012) found that by the age of 3, there is a lengthening of the coherence distances anterior-to-posterior of the brain. They state that this involves significant frequency coupling of the dorsal mediofrontal cortex to posterior regions and lengthening coherence distances in the lateral-medial direction for temporal and parietal lobes. During this age period, the brain becomes more specialized through making connections over longer distances. The P3 component in the parietal region arrives later (600–900ms) in early childhood than it does in adults (Courchesne, 1977), which is important information for researchers as they create and analyze developmental research.

EEG and ERP techniques have been successful in helping detect developmental delays in many different areas and in providing early interventions for children aged 3 to 5. Developmental ERP research suggests that there is a difference in areas of the brain underpinning face recognition in children who have autism and children who do not (Dawson and Bernier, 2013). EEG/ERP research has also been important in uncovering human development of executive control. Id est, Todd et al. (2008) reported that 4- to 6-year-olds use similar frontal networks as those employed by adults, suggesting that basic neurophysiological patterns associated with effortful control are in place as new behavioral skills are consolidating.

Elementary Age

The advent of accessible technology has altered the way children now engage in play (Bergen, Davis, & Abbitt, 2016). Also, how children are learning in schools is changing through use of one-to-one technological tools such as iPads and Chromebooks. Because new technological advances may change the ways learning occurs, they may affect both human interaction patterns and the structure of the brain. Thus, EEG and ERP studies in the field of educational neuroscience have begun to examine the effect of video games on the brain. Bergen et al. (2017) examined the difference between video games that call for an open-ended "choice" response, with no correct answer, and video games that prompt a correct/incorrect response amongst 6- to 12-year-old children. Results indicate larger brain activation responses (P3 waves) in the parietal lobe for choice conditions versus right/wrong conditions. While further research is needed to explore the elementary child's fronto-parietal system dynamics at play, this research suggests that different types of video game play will affect children's brains in various ways.

The use of EEG methods to study children's sleep is extensive, especially in relation to their effect on learning in the primary grades. Wilhelm and colleagues (2013) trained 35 children, age 8 to 11, and 37 adults in a motor sequence task involving remembering and repeating and pressing a series of lights. After a 10- to 12-hour period of wakefulness or sleep, children who had slept retained more than children who stayed awake, as well as more than adults who slept or stayed awake. While the children and adults had the same amount of rapid eye movement (REM) sleep, the children exhibited a deeper sleep pattern with greater amounts of slow-wave sleep in the Delta band (0–4Hz). This research suggests that children are developmentally primed for learning if they have sufficient sleep.

Middle Childhood

Neuroimaging studies in middle childhood looking at cortical development suggest two theories. Researchers report that during middle childhood, thinning of some cortical areas occurs alongside periods of marked development of certain cognitive functions (Casey et al., 2005; Morita, Asada, & Naito, 2016; Tau & Peterson, 2010). Sowell and colleagues (2004) suggest than an increase in language vocabulary is associated with cortical thinning in the left dorsolateral frontal and lateral parietal regions at the age of 5 to 11 years. As Figure 11.2 demonstrates, they suggest that structural brain development can have both U-shaped and linear patterns.

In a study of emotional development, Cheng, Chen, and Decety (2014) used a standardized empathy measure along with EEG/ERP methods to investigate the activation of Mu rhythms: 8–13Hz occurring over the fronto-parietal region

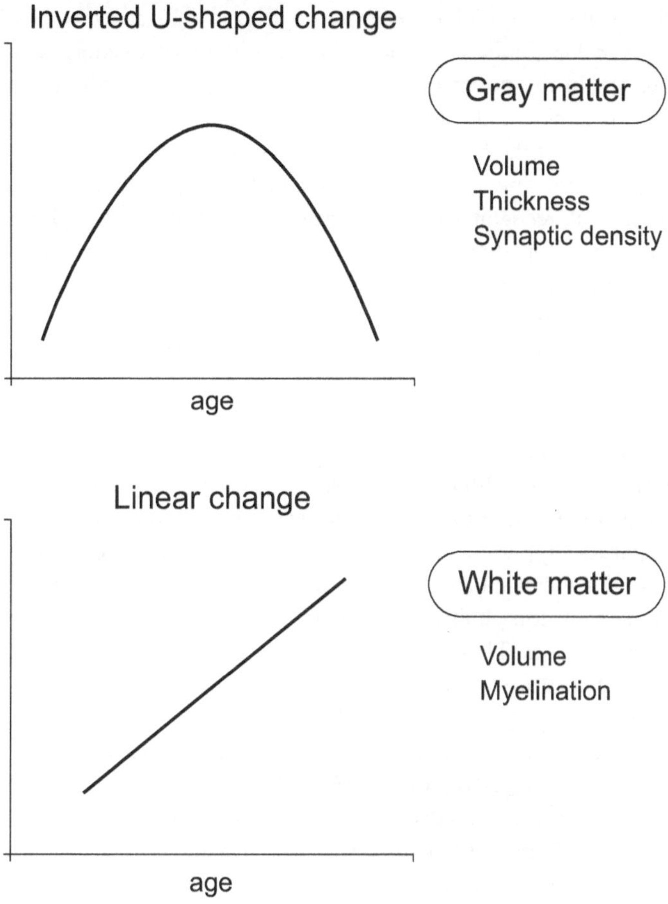

FIGURE 11.2 Structural Changes in the Brain Across Levels of Development

associated with mirror neuron perception of movement. They found an inverse relationship in empathy development and Mu frequency suppression across developmental levels of children between the ages of 5 and 12. As children aged, their levels of affective arousal (Mu) decreased while their levels of cognitive appraisal increased, coinciding with increased levels of empathy (Cheng, Chen, & Decety, 2014). The research suggests that although children in this age group feel less of the actual pain of another person, they cognitively process the events more. These developmental findings underline the importance of varied physical, socioemotional, kinesthetic and environmental experiences, and the increased role of building metacognitive reflection in the development of the middle childhood brain.

Adolescence

Results of ERP research have been important in understanding the development of the frontal lobe from adolescence to adulthood (Hogan et al., 2005). Mid-range waves such as Alpha show increases from childhood to adolescence and are often apparent in the posterior brain regions (occipital and parietal lobe areas) during resting times or during alertness. The Beta waves usually occur in the frontocentral area of the brain and are increased with excitatory activity. Gamma waves (highest frequency) have been associated with perceptual tasks requiring attention, arousal, recognition, and control of sensory processes (Bergen, 2014). EEG studies on sleep show lower predominance of frontal lobe non-rapid eye movement (NREM) that elicit Delta wave frequencies, coinciding with the late maturation of the frontal cortex (Gogtay, Giedd, & Lusk, 2004).

In a study of adolescent empathy, Mella and colleagues (2012), compared adolescent and adult ERPs during presentation of painful pictures and non-painful pictures. Their findings replicated some other ERP findings about pain related to specific ERP components, namely N110 and N340 over frontal lobes, and left posterior parietal (LPP) over the parietal. However, they also found that adolescents and adults varied in these components, with adolescents demonstrating larger amplitudes for each of the three components. Mella et al. (2012) concluded that this increased amplitude in young adolescents may reflect their lack of emotion-regulation abilities that led to more emotional arousal when they attended to pain cues. These results suggest the importance of adolescent development of self-regulatory abilities and emotional control.

Studies investigating effects of electronic media have indicated that having such media devices in children's bedrooms can have a negative effect on their sleep (Cain & Gradisar, 2010). Other EEG and neuroimaging studies have examined impacts of electronic media screen time on adolescents in the US. For example, Dworak and Wiater (2014) noted that excessive media use has been associated with impaired school performance, attention problems, and a higher risk for attention deficit hyperactivity disorder (ADHD). While adolescence may be the prime time for engagement with technology because of social media, academic requirements, and general communication during a time of identity development, research suggests that tempered use of technological devices has a less detrimental effect on the adolescent brain development.

Adulthood

EEG/ERP studies have shown particular brain regions being enlarged or diminished depending on the degree of trait or the ability of the individual (Morita, Asada, & Naito, 2016). Thus, the adult brain becomes specialized depending upon the experiences the adult has had. Daurignac, Houdé, and Jouvent (2006) found that effect in adults in a developmental study related to a Piagetian number conservation task. Participants were shown a series of screens with colored blocks both above and below a line, and they had to decide whether the number of objects above the line matched the number of objects below the line. ERP results indicated an absence of a significant P3 wave amplitude, which is typically associated with memory consolidation (Polich, 1986), yet there was a negative priming (NP) effect with the advent of a significant N2 in the frontocentral area during slow reaction time trials, suggesting that adults have cognitive traces left over from infancy and may need to inhibit some of their perceptual biases before responding to the questions. Assessment of cognitive diseases related to old age has been an area of study for ERP researchers (e.g., Polich, Ladish, & Bloom, 1990). Presently, ERP studies are being used to measure progression of Alzheimer's disease (AD). By correlating scores from a battery of psychometric tests to a slightly modified oddball paradigm with 60- to 90-year-old patients with AD, Cecchi and colleagues (2015) found significant correlations between specific subtests and P3 waves. They suggest that the ability to correlate reliable psychometric tests with neuroscientific evidence enhances doctors' abilities to diagnose the onset of AD and begin corresponding treatment.

Suggestions for Fostering Brain Development and Learning

For Families

- Families who are willing to let their typically developing children participate in EEG and ERP research studies focused on brain development issues can assist researchers in understanding brain development. Thus, they can play a role in helping increase knowledge of brain development.
- Restricting the use of screen time, especially for infants (children under 2), and monitoring time for all age groups is important. Parents should foster self-directed play and co-created experiences, especially with young children, related to motor movement, building, and design while voicing cognitive thought.
- Although children enjoy using technology-augmented media, parents should allow young children to use such media sparingly, especially during the first few years when "embodied" cognition is developing. They should monitor such media use for children of all ages, and use such media thoughtfully themselves so they can be good models for their children.

For Educators

- Educational video games, screen time, projector time, electronic whiteboard time, and other game play need to be monitored and controlled. The addictiveness of such devices is strong. Assessing the effectiveness of technology use needs to be a regular part of teachers' assessment plans.

- Attention to developmentally appropriate practices has long been a standard of appropriate teaching practices. Brain research has made it possible to understand specific naïve concepts of children and ways to assist abilities that they are capable of developing. Educators should make curricular decisions grounded in current brain research.

For Community Partners, Groups, and Policy Makers

- Funding support for researching experiential learning for young children, small communities, and society in general would provide exponential benefits for the developing young brain. Supporting or developing coordinated learning communities can be beneficial to children and parents.
- The inclusion of video games in the lives of young children and older adults has brought both promise and concern. The brain's plasticity ensures that it will change and adapt to new experiences, but because the longevity of media changes and effects on the brain have only begun to be explored, it is important that societal monitoring of such changes be continued.

Study Guide/Questions for Discussion

- Discuss how teachers can create co-constructed and community learning experiences centered around using "learning" technology.
- Select a developmental age (infant, adolescent, etc.) and read five EEG or ERP studies focused on that age level. Write a brief report outlining what has been learned about brain development from these studies and discuss implications of that information for practice.

Bibliography

American Academy of Pediatrics (AAP). (2016, October). SIDS and other sleep-related infant deaths: Updated 2016 recommendations for a safe infant sleeping environment task force on sudden infant death syndrome. *Pediatrics*, e20162938.

Andersson, A., Sanders, L. D., Karns, C. M., & Neville, H. J. (2014). Effects of age of acquisition (AoA) and proficiency on processing of syntax in 6- to 8-year-old monolingual and bilingual children: An ERP study. Paper presented at the Society for the Neurobiology of Language SNL.

Başar, E., Başar-Eroglu, C., Karakaş, S., & Schürmann, M. (2001). Gamma, alpha, delta, and theta oscillations govern cognitive processes. *International Journal of Psychophysiology, 39*(2), 241-248.

Bell, M. A., & Cuevas, K. (2012). Using EEG to study cognitive development: Issues and practices. *Journal of Cognitive Development, 13*(3), 281–294.

Bergen, D. (2014). Studying young children's cognitive and social-emotional development with ERP methodology. In O. Saracho & B. Spodek (Eds.), *Handbook of research methods in early childhood education* (Vol. 2, pp. 263–292). Greenwich, CT: Information Age.

Bergen, D., Davis, D. R., & Abbitt, J. T. (2016). *Technology play and brain development: Infancy to adolescence and future implications*. New York: Routledge.

Bergen, D., Schroer, J., Thomas, R., Zhou, X., Chou, M., & Chou, T. (2017). Child ERP responses to two stimuli types in videogame situations: Study 1 and 2 comparisons. *Journal of Research in Childhood Education, 31*(1), 160–175.

Blair, C., & Razza, R. P. (2007). Relating effortful control, executive function, and false belief understanding to emerging math and literacy ability in kindergarten. *Child Development, 78*(2), 647–663.

Blair, C., Zelazo, P. D., & Greenberg, M. T. (2005). The measurement of executive function in early childhood. *Developmental Neuropsychology, 28*(2), 561–571.

Brown, T. T., & Jernigan, T. L. (2012). Brain development during the preschool years. *Neuropsychology Review, 22*(4), 313–333

Buzsáki, G., & Wang, X. J. (2012). Mechanisms of gamma oscillations. *Annual Review of Neuroscience,* 35, 203-225.

Cain, N., & Gradisar, M. (2010). Electronic media use and sleep in school-aged children and adolescents: A review. *Sleep Medicine, 11*(8), 735-742

Casey B.J., Galvan A., Hare T.A. (2005). Changes in cerebral functional organization during cognitive development. *Current Opinion in Neurobiology, 15*(2):239–244.

Cecchi, M., Moore, D., Sadowsky, C. H., Solomon, P., Doraiswamy, M., Smith, C. D., . . . Arnold, S. E. (2015). Neuropsychological correlates of erp cognitive measures in Alzheimer's disease. *Alzheimer's & Dementia: The Journal of the Alzheimer's Association, 11*(7), P514.

Cheng, Y., Chen, C., & Decety, J. (2014). An EEG/ERP investigation of the development of empathy in early and middle childhood. *Developmental Cognitive Neuroscience,* 10, 160-169

Choisdealbha, A., & Reid, V. (2014). The developmental cognitive neuroscience of action: Semantics, motor resonance and social processing. *Experimental Brain Research, 232*(6), 1585–1597.

Courchesne, E. (1977). Event-related brain potentials: Comparison between children and adults. *Science, 197*, 589–592.

Cuevas, K., Cannon, E. N., Yoo, K., & Fox, N. (2014). The infant EEG Mu Rhythm: Methodological considerations and best practices. *Developmental Review, 34*(1), 26–43.

Daurignac, E., Houdé, O., & Jouvent, R. (2006). Negative priming in a numerical Piaget-like task as evidenced by ERP. *Journal of Cognitive Neuroscience, 18*, 730–736.

Dawson, G., & Bernier, R. (2013). A quarter century of progress on the early detection and treatment of autism spectrum disorder. *Development and Psychopathology, 25*(4pt2), 1455–1472.

Dawson, G., Carver, L., Meltzoff, A. N., Panagiotides, H., McPartland, J., & Webb, S. J. (2002). Neural correlates of face and object recognition in young children with autism spectrum disorder, developmental delay, and typical development. *Child Development, 73*(3), 700–717.

de Haan, M. (2007). Visual attention and recognition memory in infancy. Infant EEG and event-related potentials, pp. 101–143. New York: Psychology Press.

DeBoer, T., Scott, L. S., & Nelson, C. A. (2007). Event-related potentials in developmental populations. In H. Todd (Ed.), *Methodological handbook for research using event-related potentials* (pp. 263–297). Cambridge, MA: TheMIT Press.

Dworak, M., & Wiater, A. (2014). Impact of excessive media exposure on sleep and memory in children and adolescents. In *G PEO* (p. 99).

Eslinger, P. J., & Biddle, K. R. (2008). Prefrontal cortex and the maturation of executive functions, cognitive expertise, and social adaptation. In V. Anderson, R. Jacobs, & P. J. Anderson (Eds.), *Executive functions and the frontal lobes: A lifespan perspective* (pp. 299–316). Hove: Psychology Press.

Espinet, S. D., Anderson, J. E., & Zelazo, P. D. (2012). N2 amplitude as a neural marker of executive function in young children: An ERP study of children who switch versus perseverate on the dimensional change card sort. *Developmental Cognitive Neuroscience, 2*, S49–S58.

Filippi, C. A., Cannon, E. N., Fox, N. A., Thorpe, S. G., Ferrari, P. F., & Woodward, A. L. (2016). Motor system activation predicts goal imitation in 7-month-old infants. *Psychological Science, 27*(5), 675–684, 0956797616632231.

Gogtay, N., Giedd, J. N., Lusk, L., Hayashi, K. M., Greenstein, D., Vaituzis, A. C., . . . Rapoport, J. L. (2004). Dynamic mapping of human cortical development during childhood through early adulthood. *Proceedings of the National Academy of Sciences of the United States of America, 101*(21), 8174–8179.

Herrmann, C. S., Grigutsch, M., & Busch, N. A. (2005). EEG oscillations and wavelet analysis. In T. C. Handy (Ed.), *Event-related potentials: A methods handbook* (pp. 229–259). Cambridge, MA: MIT Press.

Hogan, A. M., Vargha-Khadem, F., Kirkham, F. J., & Baldeweg, T. (2005). Maturation of action monitoring from adolescence to adulthood: An ERP study. *Developmental Science, 8*(6), 525–534.

Jang, H., Kang, M., & Kim, Y. (2015). The Effect of English Extensive Reading Activities on Students Reading Proficiency and Reading Motivation. *Advanced Science and Technology Letters,* 92, 92-95.

Johnstone, T., Ores Walsh, K. S., Greischar, L. L., Alexander, A. L., Fox, A. S., Davidson, R. J., & Oakes, T. R. (2006). Motion correction and the use of motion covariates in multiple-subject fMRI analysis. *Human Brain Mapping, 27*, 779–788.

Kanai, R., & Rees, G. (2011). The structural basis of inter-individual differences in human behaviour and cognition. *Nature Reviews Neuroscience, 12*(4), 231–242.

Kuhl, P. K., Coffey-Corina, S., Padden, D., & Dawson, G. (2005). Links between social and linguistic processing of speech in preschool children with autism: behavioral and electrophysiological measures. *Developmental Science, 8*(1).

Liu, D., Sabbagh, M. A., Gehring, W. J., & Wellman, H. M. (2009). Neural correlates of children's theory of mind development. *Child Development, 80*(2), 318–326. http://doi.org/10.1111/j.1467-8624.2009.01262.x.

Lyytinen, H., Guttorm, T. K., Huttunen, T., Hämäläinen, J., Leppänen, P. H., & Vesterinen, M. (2005). Psychophysiology of developmental dyslexia: A review of findings including studies of children at risk for dyslexia. *Journal of Neurolinguistics, 18*(2), 167-195.

Mella, N., Studer, J., Gilet, A. L., & Labouvie-Vief, G. (2012). Empathy for pain from adolescence through adulthood: An event-related brain potential study. *Frontiers in Psychology, 3*, 501.

Molfese, D., & Molfese, V. (2000). The continuum of language development during infancy and childhood: Electrophysiological correlates. In C. Rovee-Collier, L. Lipsitt, & R. Reese (Eds.), *Progress in infancy research* (vol. 1, pp. 251–287). Mahwah, NJ: Erlbaum.

Morita, T., Asada, M., & Naito, E. (2016). Contribution of neuroimaging studies to understanding development of human cognitive brain functions. *Frontiers in Human Neuroscience, 10*, 464. http://doi.org/10.3389/fnhum.2016.00464.

Mulert, C., Leicht, G., Hepp, P., Kirsch, V., Karch, S., Pogarell, O., . . . McCarley, R. W. (2010). Single-trial coupling of the gamma-band response and the corresponding BOLD signal. *Neuroimage, 49*(3), 2238–2247.

Nelson C., & Monk C. (2001). The use of event-related potentials in the study of cognitive development. In Nelson, C.A. & Luciana, M. (Eds.), *Handbook of Developmental Cognitive Neuroscience*, (pp. 125-136). Cambridge, MA: MIT Press.

Pélissier, M., Krzonowski, J., & Ferragne, E. (2015, June). Effect of proficiency on subject-verb agreement processing in French learners of English: An ERP study. In *6th ISEL Conference on Experimental Linguistics.*

Pineda, J. A. (2005). The functional significance of mu rhythms: Translating "seeing" and "hearing" into "doing". *Brain Research Review, 50*, 57–68.

Pizzagalli, D. A. (2007). Electroencephalography and high-density electrophysiological source localization. *Handbook of Psychophysiology,* 3, 56-84. Oxford, UK: Cambridge University Press.

Polich, J. (1986). Normal variation of P300 from auditory stimuli. *Electroencephalography and Clinical Neurophysiology/Evoked Potentials Section, 65*(3), 236–240.

Polich, J., Ladish, C., & Bloom, F. E. (1990). P300 assessment of early Alzheimer's disease. *Electroencephalography and Clinical Neurophysiology/Evoked Potentials Section*, 77(3), 179–189.

Quiroga, R. Q., Kraskov, A., Mormann, F., Fried, I., & Koch, C. (2014). Single-cell responses to face adaptation in the human medial temporal lobe. *Neuron, 84*(2), 363-369.

Sanei, S., & Chambers, J. A. (2007). Introduction to EEG. *EEG Signal Processing*, 1-34.

Sowell E. R., Thompson P. M., Toga A.W. (2004). Mapping changes in the human cortex throughout the span of life. *Neuroscientist* 10, 372–392

Tau, G. Z., & Peterson, B. S. (2010). Normal development of brain circuits. *Neuropsychopharmacology, 35*(1), 147

Taylor, M. J., & Baldeweg, T. (2002). Application of EEG, ERP, and intracranial recordings to the investigation of cognitive functions in children. *Developmental Science, 5*, 318–334.

Todd, R. M., Lewis, M. D., Meusel, L. A., & Zelazo, P. D. (2008). The time course of social-emotional processing in early childhood: ERP responses to facial affect and personal familiarity in a Go-Nogo task. *Neuropsychologia, 46*(2), 595–613.

Ursache, A., & Noble, K. G. (2016). Neurocognitive development in socioeconomic context: Multiple mechanisms and implications for measuring socioeconomic status. *Psychophysiology, 53*(1), 71–82.

Van elk, M., Van Schie, H. T., Hunnius, S., Vesper, C., & Bekkering, H. (2008). You'll never crawl alone: Neurophysiological evidence for experience-dependent motor resonance in infancy. *Neuroimage, 43*(4), 808–814.

Wilhelm, I., Rose, M., Imhof, K. I., Rasch, B., Büchel, C., & Born, J. (2013). The sleeping child outplays the adult's capacity to convert implicit into explicit knowledge. *Nature Neuroscience, 16*(4), 391-393.

Winkler, I., Haden, G. P., Ladinig, O., Sziller, I., & Honing, H. (2008). Newborn infants detect the beat in music. *PNAS, 106*(7), 2468–2471.

Zacks, J. M. (2008). Neuroimaging studies of mental rotation: A meta-analysis and review. *Journal of Cognitive Neuroscience, 20*(1), 1–19.

12

INFLUENCE OF BRAIN RESEARCH ON CLINICAL AND EDUCATIONAL PRACTICE

Case 1 Jared's Developmental Difficulties

Jared's parents looked forward to his birth, but shortly after birth he was diagnosed with the 22q11.2 deletion syndrome (22q11.2DS), which causes a broad range of medical, health, educational, and behavioral symptoms. Jared had many medical complications, but the family had a good support system and lived about an hour from a major children's hospital with a 22q11.2DS center. Thus, he benefitted from coordinated services including a cardiac clinic to address heart problems, airway/palatal specialists, a feeding clinic, speech-language services, and genetic consultation services. Initial surgeries and medical procedures were successful, and he received early educational intervention through the local school district. Until first grade, he was involved with the hospital psychology program. The neuropsychologist there indicated that his overall cognitive functioning was within low average to average range, which was a positive finding! He had abilities in vocabulary and other verbal skills, learning and retaining rote verbal information, and phonics and word reading skills. However, weaknesses were in expressing thoughts, math/numeracy skills, ability to remember directions, working memory, visual-spatial skills, the ability to remember human faces, and difficulty understanding social situations. Behaviorally, Jared was impulsive, difficult to reward and discipline, and not adept at handling stress. He had problems with making and keeping friends. Evaluation allowed him to be identified as

Other Health Impairment (OHI), which entitled him to receive services from an intervention specialist, speech-language pathologist, occupational therapist, and school psychologist. In third grade, after social skills training, he made some friends and managed the school curriculum with extra supports. Jared had greater problems with complex academic skills (e.g., reading comprehension, written expression, and written math problem-solving). Another neuropsychological examination revealed continued problems with working memory, direction-following, understanding of visual and spatial concepts, fine motor skills, ability to process information quickly, and executive functioning (EF). These issues caused problems on the soccer field and in social relationships. His family remained positive because his health was good, the cardiac and airway problems were stable but monitored, and with the support of a psychologist in private practice, his parents were managing at home. However, Jared does not have a best friend or group of friends, and he now is asking questions about why he is different from other students and why he is not "smart." He is showing withdrawal, anxiety, and depression. Jared's attitude toward teachers remains positive, but he exhibits negativity toward school. Although he is still on the soccer team, he is not doing well personally. At the last individualized educational plan (IEP) meeting, changes to his IEP were made to address areas of identified concern. Specific evidence-based interventions in reading comprehension, written expression, and math problem-solving were identified. The school psychologist identified a social skills program and his parents found a computer-based working memory intervention prescribed by a psychologist. After consultation between his neuropsychologist and the soccer coach, Jared will stay "in the game." All are hopeful about positive changes but his progress will need to be monitored.

Understanding and Evaluating Brain-Based Interventions

Throughout history, humans have experimented with practices related to the brain, attempting to become closer to the gods, to intervene in behavior disorders, to increase brain health and power, and to understand the brain's role in guiding human behavior. Although there have been a variety of brain interventions and advances in understanding the relationship between brain development and human behavior over many years, the most remarkable leaps in understanding the brain, increasing its potential, and intervening to improve brain health have come with the advent of advanced neuroimaging techniques and clinical analysis. Henry Greely (2012), a Stanford law professor specializing in neuroethics, has noted, "neuroscience is likely to provide real direct brain interventions to treat disfavored behaviors, forcing us to decide whether, when, and how such interventions may be used" (p. 165). That comment is a reminder that the power current neuroscience affords clinicians, researchers, and educational practitioners is not without ethical dilemmas. Although these new techniques and practices can affect brain development positively, potentially improve the brain's efficiency, and ultimately cure many problems in human brain development, it does not necessarily mean that intervention is always desired or required. There have been both successful and unsuccessful brain-based interventions in the past, and although current interventions are showing promise, they have implications for professionals who use such knowledge to promote human brain development and lifelong brain functioning.

Early Brain-Based Interventions

Historically, when there have been perceived scientific advances in brain knowledge, direct brain interventions have been initiated; however, they were not always successful due to poor knowledge of potential effects of such interventions (Missios, 2004). A well-known historical example of a brain procedure that was thought to be helpful but caused greater problems was the prefrontal lobotomy. In the approximately 25-year period from its invention to its abandonment, more than 30,000 people in the United States alone were lobotomized as a treatment for a wide range of mental illnesses, without good evidence that the procedure was either safe or effective (Valenstein, 1986, Nijensohn & Goodrich, 2014). The current century has had similar issues, such as attempts to do interventions with criminals to affect their behavior. For example, Australia, Russia, South Korea, Indonesia, and the United States have implemented "chemical castration" as a mandatory punishment for certain sex offenders (Greely, 2012). Neuroscience research indicates that some less-problematic measures might help individuals who abuse drugs. Addiction is a chronic brain disease with an underlying genetic component. The growing popularity of opioids and other drugs is forcing the criminal justice system to address addiction and requiring society to ensure that scientifically based treatments that affect brain function are available (Chandler, Fletcher, & Volkow, 2009).

Implications of Brain Research for Specific Clinical and Educational Practices

Presently there are many and varied areas of brain development and health being investigated with neuroimaging techniques as well as with evidence-based interventions. Areas of study include brain interventions related to cognitive enhancement, autism intervention, dyslexia/dyscalculia, schizophrenia, Down syndrome, and 22q11.2DS.

Cognitive Enhancement

The marketing of neuropsychological interventions, cognitive enhancements, and brain-related technologies is rapidly expanding (Oullier, 2017). In 2016, a $7.6 billion market existed, and by 2020, that market is expected to be $12 billion.

New companies (e.g., Neurotech, SharpBrains) now review and monitor this burgeoning industry. The programs provide guided practice on standard sets of cognitive tasks in various domains such as working memory, language, and executive functioning (Martin et al., 2011). Widely marketed programs include BrainTrain (Burley et al., 2016), Cogmed (Spencer-Smith & Klingberg, 2015; Shinaver, Entwistle, & Soderqvist, 2014), and Jungle Memory (Alloway, Bibile, & Lau, 2013), and programs for the elderly (Martin et al., 2011). For example, in a meta-analysis of older adult programs, Kelly and colleagues (2014) found long-term cognitive training interventions increased memory retention and cognitive performance related to executive functions. Although some cognitive interventions have received generally favorable reviews and meta-analyses, outcomes also have been questioned (Melby-Lervag & Hulme, 2013). A major review of brain training research evidence (Simons et al., 2016) states that such interventions usually report improved performance on the trained tasks and modest improvement on closely related tasks, but do not improve distantly related or overall cognitive performance. The researchers also found problems in some of the reported research designs and analyses. Evaluation of such interventions should use a checklist such as that shown in Table 12.1.

Direct brain stimulation gained research traction in the early twentieth century. Noninvasive transcranial direct current stimulation (tDCS), which uses direct electrical currents to stimulate specific parts of the brain, has positively influenced cognitive functioning in healthy volunteers (Nitsche et al., 2003) and improved motor performance in volunteers at rehabilitation programs (Hummel et al., 2005).

TABLE 12.1 Checklist for Evaluating Brain-Based Cognitive Interventions

1. Is this specific intervention evidence-based? Has it been studied and found to be effective? If not, proceed with caution.
2. Has the intervention been published in a peer-reviewed journal, or studied only by the publishing company? If just studied by the company, it is not evidence-based.
3. Do the publication materials provide evidence about brain effects? Check with a school psychologist, teacher, physician, or speech-language pathologist if you have questions.
4. Does it show ways to check on an individual's progress and measure goals? If not, it will be difficult to gauge effectiveness. Measures after each session should give clear indicators.
5. If a child is successfully meeting goals, will gains generalize to classroom or behavioral success in other settings? If not, then the intervention is situation-specific and limited.
6. What are costs, time commitments, technology needed, support provided, reporting schedule, and cost guarantee? If any of these are missing, proceed with caution.
7. Does this treatment involve medical or psychological risks or invasive procedures? If so, make sure you know these before proceeding.
8. If these questions are sufficiently answered, select a program and time, a goal date, and an evaluation method. Do not proceed if these decision questions were answered negatively.

It has shown some effectiveness in treating neuropsychiatric disorders such as depression (Nitsche et al., 2009), anxiety (Shiozawa et al., 2014), attention and learning (Coffman, Clark, & Parasuraman, 2014), language learning (Flöel et al., 2008), and chronic pain relief (Mori et al., 2010). Although a tDCS device can be ordered for in-home use, this intervention has not received FDA approval.

Another area of cognitive enhancement is the use of neurofeedback to train the brain. Neurofeedback involves attempts to directly train brain functions that are not performing optimally. With EEG techniques and application of concepts of self-regulation, individuals are shown their brain "biorhythms" and attempt to train their brains (usually through playing video games) to behave appropriately. While Neuro Feedback Training (NFT) has been used clinically since the 1960s (Angelakis et al., 2007), recently it has been used primarily in clinical trials (Başar & Güntekin, 2008); Zoefel, Huster, and Herrmann (2011) and researchers report that NFT, especially of the upper Alpha band frequency, has improved cognitive performance.

It is generally accepted that the use of neuroimaging techniques such as fMRI, EEG, functional near-infrared spectroscopy (fNIRS), and structural MRI (sMRI) can monitor effectiveness of various types of cognitive training. Taya and colleagues (2015) reviewed cognitive enhancement interventions and proposed that there should be an additional level of analysis to examine biomarkers within the EEG of the individual, noting that because the brain operates as a complex network of spatially distributed regions, dedication to different functions, research, and interventions for cognitive enhancement should consider the topological architecture of the brain. Other studies have found these types of analyses may investigate increases in network global efficiency and actual network changes following working memory training (Caeyenberghs et al., 2016; Thompson, Waskom, & Gabrieli, 2016). Thus, cognitive enhancement shows promise for both research and practice.

Autism Interventions

Autism spectrum disorders (ASD) are a heterogeneous group of neurodevelopmental conditions characterized by persistent deficits in social verbal and nonverbal communication and interaction across multiple contexts (APA, 2017). While exact causes of ASD are still under debate, most research implicates both genetic and environmental factors that alter brain architecture early in life (Conti et al., 2015, NIMH, 2015). Autism is typically diagnosed by age 3; however, some characteristics may be observed around 12 months of age. According to the CDC (2016), ASD is on the rise in the US with about 1 in 68 children identified with ASD, and it is almost 4.5 times more likely to occur in males. Since the 1980s, visualization and diagnosis of ASD-related brain abnormalities have focused on structural MRI and diffusion tensor imaging (DTI) (Ismail et al., 2016). Structural MRI provides static anatomical information (such as tissue volume or gray and white matter) and functional MRI (fMRI) provides dynamic physiological information (blood flow, blood oxygen level) (Symms et al., 2004). Research comparing structural brain changes of individuals clinically diagnosed with ASD to normal functioning individuals has indicated that individuals with ASD typically have a larger cerebral cortex volume in childhood (a marker of intelligence), enlarged hippocampae (memory), smaller amygdalae volume (emotions) after childhood, and a smaller corpus collosum (left/right hemisphere connections) (Calderoni et al., 2016). According to Wolff and colleagues (2012), DTI examination of white matter fiber tracts can aid in diagnosis during ages 6 through 24 months. In contrast to cognitive enhancements where the goal is to change the brain physically through varied methods, neuroimaging technology is rarely used as a pre/post measure for behavioral interventions. However, Dawson and colleagues (2012) used EEG and ERP correlated with other behavioral measures like IQ to analyze the effectiveness of a behavioral intervention (Early Start Denver Model, ESDM) with children 18 to 30 months old. They found an increase in known neural correlates for facial recognition among the experimental group as compared with a control group. In a randomized control trial with adolescents, Van Hecke and colleagues (2015) used EEG to examine the effectiveness of a program to enhance relationship interactions (PEERS). They saw a shift in left-hemisphere frontal asymmetry in the experimental group, which they associated with more social contact ability and knowledge and reduced symptoms of ASD. Murdaugh and colleagues (2015) used resting-state fMRI to examine the effectiveness of a reading intervention program that taught the ability to form concept images as children read and heard language. They reported the experimental group showed significant post-intervention increases in reading comprehension and greater within-network functional connectivity of both Broca's and Wernicke's areas. However, although researcher and clinician knowledge of atypical formations in ASD brains are abundant, brain-based interventions remain scarce.

Dyslexia/Dyscalculia

Dyslexia is the term associated with specific learning disabilities in reading. While features of dyslexia vary individually, common characteristics include difficulty with phonemic awarenesss, phonological processing, word decoding, fluency, rate of reading, rhyming, spelling, vocabulary, comprehension, and written expression (NCLD, 2014). According to the International Dyslexia Association (2016), 85% of students who have a learning disability have primary disabilities in reading and language processing, and 15 to 20% of the general population exhibit dyslexia symptoms. Because of many factors (e.g., hereditary, epidemiology, nutrition, ADHD and other conditions), it is difficult to diagnose and elucidate cognitive causes of reading disabilities (RD) and causes of dyslexia specifically (see Shaywitz & Shaywitz, 2016). A meta-analysis conducted by Barquero, Davis, and Cutting (2014) found that RD neuroimaging studies employing fMRI and MEG reiterate most previous findings, showing under-activation in many brain locations relative to typical readers, including in the bilateral occipital regions, postcentral gyri, and inferior parietal lobes. Some studies indicate normalization can be achieved through targeted behavioral remediation emphasizing vocabulary, comprehension, word study, and fluency activities. The studies show increased responses in the inferior frontal gyrus (rhyming) and the right medial temporal cortex (word reading efficiency) (Barquero, Davis, & Cutting, 2014).

Students with Math Difficulties (MD) exhibit mathematics learning problems in one or more areas (Powell, Fuchs, & Fuchs, 2013). Although the nature of MD (present in an estimated 20% of the population) varies by student, several areas are being studied. Students with a form of MD called dyscalculia experience unusual difficulty with cardinality (i.e., telling the number of items represented in a set) and with number facts, measurement, telling time, mental math, and math problem-solving. These difficulties are attributed to inefficient counting strategies. Recent research has confirmed that there are core deficits in students' understanding of sets and in other numerocities (Butterworth, Varma, & Laurillard, 2011). Deficits in counting and cardinality can have affect progress in advanced computational domains. There is limited research examining interventions for students with MD. Researchers have found that even when intervention improves student performance, it is unclear whether cognitive and neural functioning has become more typical or whether learners developed compensatory mechanisms (Butterworth, 2011). They recommend more research is needed to gain a better understanding of intervention effectiveness. Iuculano and colleagues (2015) tested 7- to 9-year-old children over an eight-week 1:1 tutoring program. Using cognitive assessments correlated with fMRI results, they found two areas related to MD. Children with MD demonstrated pre-intervention problems with quantity, visuospatial, attention, working memory, and cognitive control processes, and showed prefrontal cortex, parietal, and ventral temporal occipital cortex effects. They report that brain overcompensation was similar to findings in RD, showing how the brain overcompensates in the areas studied for MD when giving tasks (Iuculano et al., 2015). The authors hypothesize that, due to decreased activation of areas associated with object visualization and spatial reasoning, the brain overcompensates (over-activates) in other areas, but it can return to normal functioning after successful behavioral intervention. Replication studies are needed, but the implications suggest the effectiveness of interventions and highlights the mental effort and interconnectedness of cognitive processes activated in learning mathematics.

Schizophrenia

According to the National Institute of Mental Health (2015), schizophrenia is a chronic and severe mental disorder affecting how persons think, feel, and behave. People with schizophrenia may exhibit positive (i.e., hallucinations or delusions), negative (i.e., reduced feelings of pleasure in everyday life), or cognitive symptoms (i.e., poor executive functioning or attention difficulties) beginning between the ages of 16 and 30. While causes of schizophrenia are undetermined, there are brain treatments that are useful in quieting some symptoms. Cross-sectional MRI studies show how this disease progresses in the brain and how the brain responds to treatment. Kahn et al. (2008) found that progressive brain volume loss occurred in the frontal and temporal (gray matter) areas in chronically ill patients and that habitual use of antipsychotics neither promoted nor slowed down these changes. Fusar-Poli and colleagues (2013) found, through a meta-analysis of longitudinal studies, that habitual use of antipsychotic medications is correlated with increased loss of gray matter. Whether antipsychotics cause the increase in GM loss is debatable. The most relevant current direction in treatment of schizophrenia involves attempting to change the neural circuitry of patients. Several treatments include repetitive transcranial magnetic stimulation (Sayar, Bulut, & Tarhan, 2015), transcranial direct current stimulation (Hoy et al., 2014), and deep brain stimulation. Kani et al. (2017) found through a meta-analytic review of fMRI longitudinal studies that repetitive transcranial magnetic stimulation (rTMS) and tDCS were typically effective in reducing negative symptoms and modulating networks in the frontal brain region, specifically the prefrontal cortex. Whether such treatments are the sole cause of improvements is unclear due to experiment variation, lack of follow-up, and brain area treatment specificity. Corripio and colleagues (2016) placed deep brain stimulation (DBS) electrons in the nucleus accumbens and other areas near the subgenual anterior cingulate cortex of a chronically ill middle-aged woman. Through positive and negative symptom monitoring and voltage monitoring, the researchers induced positive behavioral changes. Although results were positive, specific sites and generalizability of this research has yet to be determined.

Down Syndrome

Down syndrome is the most common chromosomal abnormality associated with intellectual disability and gets the most attention from researchers (Fidler & Nadel, 2007). Neural differences in the brain of individuals with Down syndrome can be identified as early as 22 weeks in the womb, but major differences are observed postnatally, including general reduction in fronto-occipital length, size of frontal lobes and superior temporal gyrus, and a 20–50% reduction in the cortical granular neurons (Jernigan & Bellugi, 1990). According to the CDC (2014), one in every 700 babies born in the US have Down syndrome, and the prevalence of the genetic disorder rose 30% from 1979 to 2003. Research has focused on the link between Alzheimer's and Down syndrome because nearly all individuals with Down syndrome develop Alzheimer's in their 30s (Hartley et al., 2015). Thus, the future direction in this area of research follows an interdisciplinary approach. Fidler and Nadel note that the best hope for improving such genetic disorders "lies in our ability to use all of the scientific information that is available, with developmentalists, education scientists, and brain experts collaborating" (2007, p. 269). Lott and Head (2001) reiterate suggestions to institute combination therapies, including cholinesterase inhibitors (ChEIs), antioxidants, anti-inflammatory agents, and other drugs helpful in preventing or slowing dementia in AD. While there is no cure, there is a possibility of slowing down progression of the disability. A combination of controlled supplementation with antioxidants, physical activity, and regular exercise may improve cognition and overall wellness of individuals with Down syndrome (Muchova, Zitnanova, & Durackova, 2014).

22q11.2 Microdeletion Syndrome

The 22q11.2 deletion syndrome (22q11.2DS) results from having only a small portion of chromosome 22 (McDonald-McGinn et al. (2016). The condition causes a broad range of medical, health, educational, and behavioral symptoms. The syndrome also had been known as velocardiofacial syndrome (Wang et al., 2000), featuring "velo" (airway and palatal issues), "cardio" (cardiac complications), and "facial" (common facial characteristics). It occurs in 1:300 to 1:6,000 live births, making it a common genetic disorder. Woodin and colleagues (2001) identified the neuropsychological profile of those with 22q11.2DS and noted that targeted remedial and psychosocial interventions are needed, as well as information about their cognitive and social-emotional profile, to "drive development of school techniques" (p. 38). Although guidelines for identification and practice have been written (Swillen & McDonald-McGinn, 2015), there is a need for evidence-based cognitive, educational, and social skills interventions for this group.

Neuroethical Considerations

In this century of neuroscience with neuro-research, direct brain interventions, and other treatments, neuroethics are a major consideration. Farah and colleagues note, "humanity's ability to alter its own brain function might well shape history as powerfully as the development of metallurgy in the Iron Age, mechanization in the Industrial Revolution or genetics in the second half of the twentieth century" (2004, p. 3; see also Farah, 2014). The ability of researchers and clinicians to conduct and demystify neuro-interventions places them in a unique position as gatekeepers to the real or imaginary rights of the broader society to enhance their cognitive abilities, delete unsightly memories, and treat genetic or ill-conceived biologic or psychiatric disorders. They have a great responsibility to inform each other, clinicians, educators, judges, politicians, and the public about real and potential dangers of pursuing such cutting-edge research. Another ethical aspect of research involving direct brain interventions focuses on interventions for incarcerated individuals with psychiatric disorders. While most professionals support limited use of techniques like DBS (Hübner & White, 2016), it is important to note that the jury is still out on this issue, and the court system, as well as the court of public opinion, will have to take a stand regarding the level of freedom or mental integrity that incarcerated individuals may own (Craig, 2016).

Implications of Brain Research for Advocacy of Excellence in Clinical and Educational Practice

- Current brain-based interventions rely on assertions that the present neuroimaging techniques are appropriate for exploring brain activity and determining learning and behavior deficits. When behavioral interventions are not successful, parents, educators, and practitioners should explore diagnosis and treatment with neuroimaging techniques.
- Brain neuroplasticity suggests that effective neuro-oriented or behavioral intervention may change the structure or functioning of the brain. Learning and behavior effects must be observed and "normal" brain functioning identified.
- Parents, educators, clinicians, and other practitioners must value the ability of the brain to develop new neural pathways and adapt to new cognitive demands. A neuro-growth mindset can promote positive interactions between adults and children and result in improvements in learning.
- Because neuroimaging techniques and analysis have advanced greatly over the past five to ten years, recent findings are likely to create further advances. Thus, educators, researchers, and clinicians should remain current on brain-based knowledge and intervention methods.

Study Guide/Questions for Discussion

- Plan a talk about the role of interdisciplinary perspectives in researching and implementing brain-based interventions and explain how multiple perspectives increase the chances of making substantive positive change in human lives.
- Research an area that uses a multidisciplinary intervention approach or where a multidisciplinary approach could be used. Discuss the pros and cons of the approach.
- Many brain-based interventions are not known or accessible to the public. List the ethical responsibilities of society in creating, funding, and publicizing such methods.

Bibliography

Alloway, T. P., Bibile, V., & Lau, G. (2013). Computerized working memory training: Can it lead to gains in cognitive skills in students? *Computers in Human Behavior*, *29*(3), 632–638.

American Psychological Association. (2017). Retrieved from www.apa.org/topics/autism/.

Angelakis, E., Stathopoulou, S., Frymiare, J. L., Green, D. L., Lubar, J. F., & Kounios, J. (2007). EEG neurofeedback: A brief overview and an example of peak alpha frequency training for cognitive enhancement in the elderly. *The Clinical Neuropsychologist*, *21*(1), 110–129.

Barquero, L. A., Davis, N., & Cutting, L. E. (2014). Neuroimaging of reading intervention: A systematic review and activation likelihood estimate meta-analysis. *PLOS One*, *9*(1), 1–16.

Başar, E., & Güntekin, B. (2008). A review of brain oscillations in cognitive disorders and the role of neurotransmitters. *Brain Research*, *1235*, 172–193.

Burley, C.V., Bailey, D. M., Marley, C. J., & Lucas, S. J. (2016). Brain train to combat brain drain; focus on exercise strategies that optimize neuroprotection. *Experimental Physiology*, *101*(9), 1178–1184.

Butterworth, B. (2010). Foundational numerical capacities and the origins of dyscalculia. *Trends in Cognitive Sciences*, *14*(12), 534–541.

Butterworth, B., Varma, S., & Laurillard, D. (2011). Dyscalculia: From brain to education. *Science*, *332*(6033), 1049–1053.

Caeyenberghs, K., Metzler-Baddeley, C., Foley, S., & Jones, D. K. (2016). Dynamics of the human structural connectome underlying working memory training. *Journal of Neuroscience*, *36*(14), 4056–4066.

Calderoni, S., Billeci, L., Narzisi, A., Brambilla, P., Retico, A., & Muratori, F. (2016). Rehabilitative interventions and brain plasticity in autism spectrum disorders: Focus on MRI-based studies. *Frontiers in Neuroscience*, *10*, 1–7.

Centers for Disease Control. (2014). Retrieved February 21, 2017, from www.cdc.gov/ncbddd/birthdefects/downsyndrome/data.html, page last reviewed October 21, 2014; page last updated October 21, 2014.

Centers for Disease Control. (2016). Retrived from February 7, 2017, www.cdc.gov/ncbddd/autism/data.html, page last reviewed September 26, 2016; page last updated July 11, 2016.

Chandler, R. K., Fletcher, B. W., & Volkow, N. D. (2009). Treating drug abuse and addiction in the criminal justice system: Improving public health and safety. *JAMA*, *301*(2), 183–190.

Coffman, B. A., Clark, V. P., & Parasuraman, R. (2014). Battery powered thought: Enhancement of attention, learning, and memory in healthy adults using transcranial direct current stimulation. *Neuroimage*, *85*, 895–908.

Conti, E., Calderoni, S., Marchi, V., Muratori, F., Cioni, G., & Guzzetta, A. (2015). The first 1000 days of the autistic brain: A systematic review of diffusion imaging studies. *Frontiers in Human Neuroscience*, *9*, art. no. 159.

Corripio, I., Sarró, S., McKenna, P. J., Molet, J., Álvarez, E., Pomarol-Clotet, E., & Portella, M. J. (2016). Clinical improvement in a treatment-resistant patient with schizophrenia treated with deep brain stimulation. *Biological Psychiatry*, *80*(8), e69–e70.

Craig, J. N. (2016). Incarceration, direct brain intervention, and the right to mental integrity—a reply to Thomas Douglas. *Neuroethics*, *9*(2), 107–118.

Dawson, G., Jones, E. J., Merkle, K., Venema, K., Lowy, R., Faja, S., . . . Smith, M. (2012). Early behavioral intervention is associated with normalized brain activity in young children with autism. *Journal of the American Academy of Child & Adolescent Psychiatry*, *51*(11), 1150–1159.

Farah, M. J. (2014). The unknowns of cognitive enhancement: Can science and policy catch up with practice? *Science*, *350*(6259), 379–380.

Farah, M. J., Illes, J., Cook-Deegan, R., Gardner, H., Kandel, E., King, P., . . . Wolpe, P. R. (2004). Neurocognitive enhancement: What can we do and what should we do? *Nature Reviews Neuroscience*, *5*(5), 421–425.

Fidler, D. J., & Nadel, L. (2007). Education and children with Down syndrome: Neuroscience, development, and intervention. *Developmental Disabilities Research Reviews*, *13*(3), 262–271.

Flöel, A., Rösser, N., Michka, O., Knecht, S., & Breitenstein, C. (2008). Noninvasive brain stimulation improves language learning. *Journal of Cognitive Neuroscience, 20*(8), 1415–1422.

Fusar-Poli, P., Smieskova, R., Kempton, M. J., Ho, B. C., Andreasen, N. C., & Borgwardt, S. (2013). Progressive brain changes in schizophrenia related to antipsychotic treatment? A meta-analysis of longitudinal MRI studies. *Neuroscience & Biobehavioral Reviews, 37*(8), 1680–1691.

Greely, H. T. (2012). Direct brain interventions to "treat" disfavored human behaviors: Ethical and social issues. *Clinical Pharmacology and Therapeutics, 91*(2), 163.

Hartley, D., Blumenthal, T., Carrillo, M., DiPaolo, G., Esralew, L., Gardiner, K., . . . Lott, I. (2015). Down syndrome and Alzheimer's disease: Common pathways, common goals. *Alzheimer's & Dementia, 11*(6), 700–709.

Hoy, K. E., Arnold, S. L., Emonson, M. R., Daskalakis, Z. J., & Fitzgerald, P. B. (2014). An investigation into the effects of tDCS dose on cognitive performance over time in patients with schizophrenia. *Schizophrenia Research, 155*(1), 96–100.

Hübner, D., & White, L. (2016). Neurosurgery for psychopaths? An ethical analysis. AJOB *Neuroscience,* 7(3), 140-149.

Hummel, F., Celnik, P., Giraux, P., Floel, A., Wu, W. H., Gerloff, C., & Cohen, L. G. (2005). Effects of non-invasive cortical stimulation on skilled motor function in chronic stroke. *Brain, 128*(3), 490–499.

International Dyslexia Association. (2016). *How widespread is dyslexia?* Retrieved February 8, 2017, from https://dyslexiaida.org/how-widespread-is-dyslexia/.

Ismail, M. M., Keynton, R. S., Mostapha, M. M., ElTanboly, A. H., Casanova, M. F., Gimel'farb, G. L., & El-Baz, A. (2016). Studying autism spectrum disorder with structural and diffusion magnetic resonance imaging: a survey. *Frontiers in Human Neuroscience,* 10.

Iuculano, T., Rosenberg-Lee, M., Richardson, J., Tenison, C., Fuchs, L., Kaustubh, S., . . . Menon, V. (2015). Cognitive tutoring induces widespread neuroplasticity and remediates brain function in children with mathematical learning disabilities. *Nature Communication, 6*, 1–10.

Jernigan, T. L., & Bellugi, U. (1990). Anomalous brain morphology on magnetic resonance images in Williams syndrome and Down syndrome. *Archives of Neurology, 47*(5), 529–533.

Kahn, R. S., Fleischhacker, W. W., Boter, H., Davidson, M., Vergouwe, Y., Keet, I. P., . . . Hummer, M. (2008). Effectiveness of antipsychotic drugs in first-episode schizophrenia and schizophreniform disorder: An open randomised clinical trial. *The Lancet, 371*(9618), 1085–1097.

Kani, A. S., Shinn, A. K., Lewandowski, K. E., & Ongur, D. (2017). Review article: Converging effects of diverse treatment modalities on frontal cortex in schizophrenia: A review of longitudinal functional magnetic resonance imaging studies. *Journal of Psychiatric Research, 84*, 256–276.

Kelly, M. E., Loughrey, D., Lawlor, B. A., Robertson, I. H., Walsh, C., & Brennan, S. (2014). The impact of cognitive training and mental stimulation on cognitive and everyday functioning of healthy older adults: A systematic review and meta-analysis. *Ageing Research Reviews, 15*, 28–43.

Lott, I. T., & Head, E. (2001). Down syndrome and Alzheimer's disease: A link between development and aging. *Mental Retardation and Developmental Disabilities Research Reviews,* 7(3), 172–178.

Martin, M. (2011). Cutadapt removes adapter sequences from high-throughput sequencing reads. *EMBnet Journal, 17*(1), 10.

McDonald-McGinn, D. M., Sullivan, K. E., Marino, B., Philip, N., Swillen, A., & Vorstman, J. A. S. (2016). 22q11.2 deletion syndrome. *Nature Reviews Disease Primers, 1*, 15071. https://doi.org/10.1038/nrdp.2015.71. PMID: 27189754.

Melby-Lervåg, M., & Hulme, C. (2013). Is working memory training effective? A meta-analytic review. *Developmental Psychology, 49*(2), 270.

Missios, S. (2004). Hippocrates, Galen, and the uses of trepanation in the ancient classical world. *Neurosurgery Focus, 23*(1), 1–8.

Mori, F., Codecà, C., Kusayanagi, H., Monteleone, F., Buttari, F., Fiore, S., . . . & Centonze, D. (2010). Effects of anodal transcranial direct current stimulation on chronic neuropathic pain in patients with multiple sclerosis. *The Journal of Pain, 11*(5), 436-442.

Muchova, J., Zitnanova, I., & Durackova, Z. (2014). Oxidative stress and down syndrome. Do antioxidants play a role in therapy? *Physiological Research, 63*(5), 535.

Murdaugh, D. L., Maximo, J. O., & Kana, R. K. (2015). Changes in intrinsic connectivity of the brain's reading network following intervention in children with autism. *Human Brain Mapping, 36*, 2965–2979.

NCLD. (2014). *The state of learning disabilities: Facts, trends and emerging issues*. Retrieved February 8, 2017, from www.ncld.org/wp-content/uploads/2014/11/2014-State-of-LD.pdf.

Nijensohn, D. E., & Goodrich, I. (2014). Psychosurgery: Past, present, and future, including prefrontal lobotomy and Connecticut's contribution. *Connecticut Medicine, 78*(8), 453–463.

NIMH. (2015). *Autism spectrum disorder*. Bethesda, MD: Office of Science Policy.

Nitsche, M. A., Boggio, P. S., Fregni, F., & Pascual-Leone, A. (2009). Treatment of depression with Transcranial Direct Current Stimulation (tDCS): A review. *Experimental Neurology, 219*(1), 14–19.

Nitsche, M. A., Liebetanz, D., Antal, A., Lang, N., Tergau, F., & Paulus, W. (2003). Modulation of cortical excitability by weak direct current stimulation—technical, safety and functional aspects. *Supplements to Clinical Neurophysiology, 56*, 255–276.

Oullier, O. (2017, May 2). This is your brain on business. *Fortune*. Retrieved from http://fortune.com/2017/05/02/neurotechnology-brainstorm-health-oullier/.

Pol, H. E. H., & Kahn, R. S. (2008). What happens after the first episode? A review of progressive brain changes in chronically ill patients with schizophrenia. *Schizophrenia Bulletin, 34*(2), 354–366.

Powell, S. R., Fuchs, L. S., & Fuchs, D. (2013). Reaching the mountaintop: Addressing the common core standards in mathematics for students with mathematics difficulties. *Learning Disabilities Research & Practice, 28*(1), 38-48

Sayar, G. H., Bulut, H., & Tarhan, N. (2015). Use of repetitive transcranial magnetic stimulation in treatment of negative symptoms of schizophrenia. *Journal of Neurology, Neurological Science and Disorders, 1*(1), 017, 21, 017.

Shaywitz, S. E., & Shaywitz, B. A. (2016, April 15). Reading disability and the brain. *On Developing Readers: Readings from Educational Leadership (EL Essentials)*, p. 146.

Shinaver III, C. S., Entwistle, P. C., & Söderqvist, S. (2014). Cogmed WM training: Reviewing the reviews. *Applied Neuropsychology: Child, 3*(3), 163–172.

Shiozawa, P., Leiva, A. P. G., Castro, C. D. C., da Silva, M. E., Cordeiro, Q., Fregni, F., & Brunoni, A. R. (2014). Transcranial direct current stimulation for generalized anxiety disorder: A case study. *Biological Psychiatry, 75*(11), e17–e18.

Simons, D. J., Boot, W. R., Charness, N., Gathercole, S. E., Chabris, C. F., Hambrick, D. Z., & Stine-Morrow, E. A. (2016). Do "brain-training" programs work? *Psychological Science in the Public Interest, 17*(3), 103–186.

Spencer-Smith, M., & Klingberg, T. (2015). Benefits of a working memory training program for inattention in daily life: A systematic review and meta-analysis. *PLoS One, 10*(3), e0119522.

Swillen, A., & McDonald-McGinn, D. (2015). Developmental trajectories in 22q11. 2 deletion syndrome. *American Journal of Medical Genetics Part C: Seminars in Medical Genetics, 169*(2), 172–181.

Symms, M., Jäger, H. R., Schmierer, K., & Yousry, T. A. (2004). A review of structural magnetic resonance neuroimaging. *Journal of Neurology, Neurosurgery & Psychiatry, 75*(9), 1235–1244.

Taya, F., Sun, Y., Babiloni, F., Thakor, N., & Bezerianos, A. (2015). Brain enhancement through cognitive training: A new insight from brain connectome. *Frontiers in Systems Neuroscience, 9*(44), 1–19.

Thompson, T. W., Waskom, M. L., & Gabrieli, J. D. (2016). Intensive working memory training produces functional changes in large-scale frontoparietal networks. *Journal of Cognitive Neuroscience, 28*(4), 575–588.

U. S. Department of Health and Human Services, National Institutes of Health, National Institute of Mental Health. (2016, February). *NIMH mental health information.* Retrieved from www.nimh.nih.gov/health/topics/schizophrenia/index.shtml.

Valenstein, E. S. (1986). *Great and desperate cures: The rise and decline of psychosurgery and other radical treatments for mental illness.* New York: Basic Books.

Van Hecke, A.V., Stevens, S., Carson, A. M., Karst, J. S., Dolan, B., Schohl, K., . . . Brockman, S. (2015). Measuring the plasticity of social approach: A randomized controlled trial of the effects of the PEERS intervention on EEG asymmetry in adolescents with autism spectrum disorders. *Journal of Autism and Developmental Disorders, 45*(2), 316–335.

Wang, P. P., Woodin, M. F., Kreps-Falk, R., & Moss, E. M. (2000). Research on behavioral phenotypes: Velocardiofacial syndrome (deletion 22q11. 2). *Developmental Medicine & Child Neurology, 42*(6), 422–427.

Wolff, J. J., Gu, H., Gerig, G., Elison, J. T., Styner, M., Gouttard, S., . . . Evans, A. C. (2012). Differences in white matter fiber tract development present from 6 to 24 months in infants with autism. *American Journal of Psychiatry, 169*(6), 589–600.

Woodin, M., Wang, P. P., Aleman, D., McDonald-McGinn, D., Zackai, E., & Moss, E. (2001). Neuropsychological profile of children and adolescents with the 22q11.2 microdeletion. *Genetics in Medicine, 3*(1), 34–39.

Zoefel, B., Huster, R. J., & Herrmann, C. S. (2011). Neurofeedback training of the upper alpha frequency band in EEG improves cognitive performance. *Neuroimage, 54*(2), 1427–1431.

13

EVALUATING PROFESSIONAL PRACTICES FROM A BRAIN RESEARCH PERSPECTIVE

As preceding chapters have shown, although there are no definitive answers, hypotheses and recommendations from brain development research may be useful for educators, clinicians, and other social service professionals. This chapter reviews implications for professional practice and suggests methods of advocacy to foster optimal brain development.

Implications of Brain Research for Professional Practice

Many practices that professionals support are based on human development principles and observations of effective practice. These practices now may be informed by research on brain growth and neurological development. This section evaluates common practices in the light of current brain research.

Art and Music Early Experiences

The effects of early exposure to art and music on brain growth and neurological development have been the focus of some study. In a review, Hallam (2010) concluded that extensive music training and performance over long periods supports positive brain development in fine motor coordination, spatial reasoning, and possibly perceptual skills. Moreno and colleagues (2011) found that child music training may enhance executive functioning; Wan and Schlau (2010) note that there may be lifelong brain effects of music experiences; and Summa-Chadwick (2009) suggests that music protocol training is related to neurological benefits for children with special needs. However, playing classical music to infants to improve their cognitive abilities (see Omaha World Herald, 1999) is not supported by research. Art and music activities, especially long term, may enhance synaptogenesis in certain brain structures and affect brain pruning processes. Zeki (2001) suggests that extensive research is needed on the neural basis of artistic creativity. Until longitudinal research is available, early exposure to *specific* art and music experiences (e.g., Mozart) does not "guarantee" that children will be more adept at related skills.

Computers, Electronic Tablets, and Other "Smart" Toys

The explosion of technology-augmented toys and other electronic devices has raised questions about long-term effects on brain development. Short-term studies of potential cognitive effects of children's computer use report that metacognition may be enhanced with programming experiences (e.g., Miller, Church, & Trexler, 2000) and child learning may be improved through the use of electronic tablets (Lee, 2015). However, long-term effects have not been studied. Informal observations and narrative accounts of high computer game use suggest that cognitive "multitasking" may be enhanced and social skills may develop in different ways (e.g., electronic "friends" supplanting face-to-face ones). Whether behavioral changes are reflected in brain structures or neurological functions is unclear. Little is known about young children's recent immersion in technology-augmented devices, such as "smart" toys and electronic tablets. Virtual toys and devices may provide more stimulation to certain brain areas and less to other areas stimulated more by real environment interactions. "Enactive cognition," which is facilitated by physical interactions with real-world objects, may be less developed while "iconic" and "symbolic" cognition may be enhanced (Bruner, 1964). Also, "mirror neuron" development and face-to-face social interactions may be affected by pervasive interaction with virtual worlds, especially if it reduces parent-infant face-to-face social interactions (see Bergen, Davis, & Abbitt, 2016).

Information from a range of sources (e.g., reading, discussions, outdoor experiences) as well as from electronically augmented sources is warranted, and real as well as virtual friends are needed. Long-term brain research to investigate the brain development of those who use technology media extensively should be initiated. Whether a "technological brain" is adaptive for contemporary culture is a matter of debate (Courage et al., 2015). Because information is lacking on brain structural changes and neurological differences fostered in new technology environments, the use of such media should be monitored and efforts should be made to encourage human brain engagement in all types of knowledge construction, including physically active ones.

Cooperative Learning

The cooperative learning literature (e.g., Johnson & Johnson, 1994; Slavin, 1995) made a strong case for its efficacy for social and cognitive development. Evidence from brain research indicates that emotion and cognition are connected and social attachments may affect brain structures and functions. However, research has not examined how cooperative learning directly affects brain structural growth or neurological development. Research has shown effects of cooperative learning for children with problems in social-emotional and cognitive functioning, such as those with autism or ADHD (e.g., Grey Honan et al., 2007; Zentall, Kuester, & Craig, 2011). Providing such learning experiences may stimulate synaptogenesis in social-emotional networks in the brain. Recent research on the effectiveness of cooperative learning in secondary schools has supported its value as a learning method (see Kyndt et al., 2013; Zakaria et al., 2013).

Critical Periods for Timing Certain Educational Experiences

An assumption made after neuroimaging research described the rapid occurrence of synaptogenesis in infancy was that there were brief critical periods for certain aspects of brain growth and neurological development. While there are some critical periods in prenatal brain growth and neurological development (e.g., cortical migration), most researchers use the term "sensitive periods" to suggest that certain aspects of brain growth and neurological development are stronger at some periods. However, the time periods are broad rather than brief (Knudsen, 2004). Humans do not "bond" emotionally in a brief critical period right after birth but develop emotional attachment over the first year of life. Comprehension of language has a shorter sensitive period than language expression, which can develop through the early childhood years. Motor development also follows a sensitive but not a critical time schedule. Research on effects of preschool enrichment on long-term development suggests that during this early age period when synaptic development is at its peak, experientially rich, safe, and challenging environments that facilitate all aspects of growth may have long-term effects on brain development and later life behaviors and abilities. Likewise, adolescence may be a sensitive period for issues related to memory, social stress, and drug use (Fuhrmann, Knoll, & Blakemore, 2015). However, the brain's plasticity makes the idea of short critical periods for brain growth and neurological development unlikely. Educators and other professionals should not "give up" on any child just because that child did not have certain experiences during an optimum sensitive period. The brain's ability to make structural and functional changes when new experiences are encountered is evident throughout the lifespan (see Bailey et al., 2001).

Developmentally Appropriate Early Childhood Practice

The early childhood field has stressed the importance of developmentally appropriate experiences designed for children's cognitive, motor, sensory, social-emotional, and language development. Brain research information seems compatible with current early education practice. The amazing plasticity of the brain and the phenomenal growth in synapses during the early years suggest that, with adult scaffolding, young children may be capable of learning more than the information that is traditionally part of the early childhood curriculum. Nevertheless, vigorously marketed "brain-based curricula" are not based on applied brain research. Experiences of children from deprived backgrounds should be expanded in developmentally appropriate ways to facilitate synaptogenesis, however. Active learning experiences and wide choices of experiences are in line with present knowledge of brain growth and neurological development.

Emotional Development as an Educational Goal

Brain research has made changes in the simplistic "triune" brain model, which hypothesized that emotions were in the "mammalian" brain (i.e., the limbic system). It is now known that there are strong interactive linkages between structures that generate emotions and structures that recognize and control emotions, which are primarily in the "neomammalian" brain (i.e., the cerebral cortex). Although infants show and recognize most emotions, as children's brains mature, they gain the capacity to label, categorize, and interpret emotions, and these processes affect basic emotions and cognitive, language, and social meanings. Research on episodic memory indicates that best-remembered events are those embedded in strong emotions (both positive and negative), suggesting that learning should be embedded in positive emotional contexts (Mercer, 2013). Although there are a limited number of brain imaging studies related to emotion-based learning, it is likely that brain research supports awareness of the importance of emotions in learning (Blakemore & Robbins, 2012; Crone & Dahl, 2012; Spear, 2013).

Fine/Gross Motor Development as an Educational Goal

Studies of motor and sensory brain areas indicate that actions requiring precise movement and motor coordination take up more space in the motor cortex than do broader but less demanding activities. For example, the motor cortex allots more space to actions of the tongue and lips than to the foot. Children require motor action both for its own sake and for its ability to enhance all learning modes. Learning to inhibit motor activity is also important, especially for development of certain areas of the brain, and there is complexity in the interactions among various brain areas that are required to inhibit or to coordinate actions. Children should have multisensory input and be motorically active while learning, but no specific gross motor movements (e.g., crawling) or movement routines (e.g., exercising the right hemisphere by left-side body movements) are supported by brain research. Research using neuroimaging does show that a "reading circuit" may be activated across the inferior frontal gyrus, the fusiform gyrus, and the anterior cingulate when fine motor skills are involved in learning literacy skills (James & Englehardt, 2012; Kersey & James, 2013). Professionals should provide a balance of sedentary, active body, and gross/fine motor experiences so that "embodied cognition" continues to be promoted.

First and Second Language Learning

There is presently interest in providing earlier second language experiences and research indicates that when more than one language is learned in early childhood, there are changes in the brain's electrical activity, in the location of this activity within the brain, and in the structure of the learners' brains (Osterhout et al., 2008). Because discrimination and reproduction of non-native-language phonemes diminishes with age, second (or third) language learning should be initiated before or at least by middle childhood. Although the ability to learn another language throughout life exists because of the brain's plasticity, it is more difficult at later ages. Thus, it is counterproductive to reserve first teaching of foreign languages to middle school or high school when the optimum time for learning a second language is earlier. Also, because speakers of multiple rather than only one language appear to have brain advantages, professionals should encourage children to remain fluent in their native language as they also become speakers of the language of the common culture.

Health and Nutrition Education

Evidence from prenatal and infancy brain research is clear about the importance of adequate nutrition and good health practices (e.g., avoiding drug use). Because brain size and weight is primarily completed in early childhood and the young brain uses such a large proportion of body energy, it is likely to suffer from deprivation of nutrition or effects of teratogenic substances or disease during that period. Professionals and parents should be aware of the importance of early nutrition and health (including prenatally) and stress the importance of lifelong nutrition and healthful practice. As of this time, although having health-promoting diets is warranted, there is no clear evidence that certain foods can especially enhance brain growth and development.

Inclusion of Diverse Populations

One of the major rationales for inclusion of children with disabilities into classrooms with other children is that they will gain more relevant social experiences and cognitive stimulation than they will receive in separate "resource room" programs. While brain research does not speak directly to this issue, inferences might be drawn on both sides of the inclusion debate. On the side of inclusion, exposure to a wider range of experiences, such as those encountered in a regular classroom, and being challenged at their highest levels of ability by doing as much of the "regular" work as is possible, may enhance children's synaptic growth and neurological development. Conversely, being in a classroom with a small group of children and having intensive learning experiences might also strengthen synaptic connections in functional areas. Brain research is providing information about brain development in children with learning disabilities, autism spectrum disorder, attention deficit hyperactivity, and other disorders. However, presently there is no strong research evidence as to one best educational environment for such children. Each child's needs and abilities should be the standard for deciding on what level of inclusion is best.

Intervention Practices

Specific intervention practices most effective with children with various disabilities are still debated and proponents of certain approaches do not agree. Early intervention research has confirmed that rich early experiences seem to benefit most children. Specific intervention practices promoted by special educators, physical and occupational therapists, and other professionals working with children who have disabilities (e.g., sensory integration) are not yet clearly supported by evidence from brain research, although proponents of certain approaches have made claims about such neurological effects for many years. Research now being conducted may result in more definitive answers regarding interventions. Practices that have been shown to be supportive of brain development for other children should be provided for these children also.

Left Brain/Right Brain Teaching Strategies

While brain research has delineated differences in structures and functions of the two brain hemispheres and in the corpus callosum, recommended educational practices to teach to the left brain or right brain have far exceeded research evidence. Having experiences that strengthen all areas of the brain is most effective and there should be no gender differences in experiences. One value of "right-left brain" discussions has been the importance of broadening experiences to include those purportedly more allied to "left brain" (logic/language) and "right brain" (e.g., the arts, social-emotional, spatial). That is, "whole brain" experiences probably are best. Because the brain is an integrated entity, children should not be encouraged to think of themselves as "right-brained" or "left-brained" because the brain operates with "wholeness" in all individuals. The educational aim should be to help children build skills in all areas.

Memory Teaching Strategies

Numerous theories have been posited to explain memory and many types have been described. It is unclear, however, whether all brain areas involved in memory have been identified and exactly how memories are generated. Studies suggest that many brain structures are involved in memory and that neurological connections hold memory as well. Helping children learn memory strategies that call upon varied functions of the brain (e.g., visual, auditory, motor, emotional) can enhance memory capabilities and strengthen synaptic connections for learning. It is likely that the more memory links that can be "hard-wired" into the brain before synaptic pruning begins, the greater memory abilities in general will be. Brain processes governing working memory are of vital importance for learning (Kharitonova et al., 2015). Memory can be assisted through instructional strategies (Dehn, 2011; Swanso, 2016) as well as with evidence-based computer programs at home or school (Holmes & Gathercole, 2014; Peijnenborgh et al., 2016). Families can gain assistance regarding such strategies from school psychologists, pediatricians, or pediatric neuropsychologists.

Metacognitive Teaching Strategies

An even greater mystery is that of metacognition, which is the ability to think about one's own thinking. Metacognition is one aspect of "consciousness" and thus, presently, there are no answers to how or where it occurs. Research on the frontal lobe has pointed to this site as being involved in thinking processes related to metacognition, such as predicting, analyzing, and evaluating experiences. Answers to these questions may be found in research on the brains (especially the frontal lobes) of individuals who seem to lack some of these skills. Even if the precise site of metacognitive strategies in the brain is unclear, it is especially important for educators and other professionals to facilitate children's development of metacognitive strategies because they provide the basis for formal operations and other abstract thought. The true mystery of metacognition will not be solved until brain researchers understand what is involved in consciousness.

Multiple Intelligences Teaching Strategies

Gardner's multiple intelligences theory (Gardner, 2011) has been promoted as an educational strategy and curricula have been devised based on the tenets of the theory. Some models advise having experiences that "exercise all" intelligences while others focus on teaching to each student's supposed intellectual strengths. While different parts of the brain are more active during certain types of learning experiences (e.g., visual and language areas active in reading), there are no studies showing one-to-one correspondence between parts of the brain and certain types of intelligence. Gardner has expressed concern that interpretations of his theory have focused on the "learning styles" approach. Until more is known about neurological bases for multiple intelligence theory, children should probably have opportunities to exercise all modes of intelligence and to gain mastery of as many as possible, and they should not be confined to one "learning style."

New Math and Old Math

Although proponents of some "brain-based" curricula stress that it helps children learn mathematical concepts more effectively, applying brain research to the teaching of mathematics requires a big leap. Certain aspects of mathematics involve use of spatial skills while others are primarily related to symbol understanding and use of algorithms. Manipulating mathematical quantities with concrete objects and with symbol systems are vastly different. Ordering geometric patterns of shapes/sizes involves different areas of the brain than memorizing the multiplication tables. Recent "new" math emphasis on critical thinking and problem-solving skills may enhance frontal lobe development while "old" math attention to learning algorithms and number facts may further development of brain areas activated by memory tasks. It is probably the case that giving children exposure to many varied math learning methods may give the greatest stimulation to the brain. Although no definitive research linking specific areas of brain growth and neurological development to certain mathematical teaching methods is presently in existence, playful and active opportunities to use mathematical thinking is important.

Oral Language and Emerging Literacy

The earliest years of life involve development of oral language, and emerging literacy skills begin to develop even in late infancy, especially in environments where parents interact in early book "reading." However, no brain research supports specific teaching of literacy skills in infancy or shows evidence that brain development is significantly altered by direct teaching of language/literacy at early ages. Language expression has a wide "range of normality" in development. One factor beneficial for later literacy skills is having a wide vocabulary and strong language proficiency so parent/child talk is very important. Much emphasis is presently being put on emerging literacy during the age 3 to 5 period, and there is some research that suggests this type of literacy is essential for later reading excellence. Presently, psychological and educational research supports efforts to foster emerging literacy through extensive language and literacy experiences without resorting to research linking it to specific brain areas.

Play in the Curriculum

Most developmental theorists and early educators note that play provides a range of stimulating experiences likely to foster optimum synaptogenesis. Although research shows that cognitive, social-emotional, and motor skills are enhanced by play, the importance of play has not been related to brain research except in a few instances, such as in Panksepp's (1998) speculations drawn from studies of ADHD that play may aid maturation of the frontal cortex. Play does serve important functions that can be hypothetically related to brain research. It is highly motivating to young children and they are inclined to repeat enjoyable activities in play. The repetition and elaboration of "practice play" may strengthen synaptic connections and create levels of mastery that contribute to neurological development. Pretend play has long been related to exercise of brain functions such as symbolic representation, imagination, social-emotional control, and language use. Game playing involves qualities of both practice and pretend play, and fosters skills of prediction, self-regulation, and motor coordination. Sylwester noted (1995) that the frontal lobe's "extra" capacity, useful for problem-solving in emergencies, is exercised in non-emergency times by creating problems to solve in imaginary and playful realms. Thus, while there is no brain research evidence linking play development to specific areas of neurological development, professionals and parents who give opportunities for play are likely to be supporting brain functioning.

Pro-social and Social Skill Development as Educational Goals

Problems with social interaction often have been noted in children who exhibit neurodevelopmental disorders or specific brain trauma. Psychological research has discussed positive behavioral support (PBS) and social skills training (e.g., Gardner & Hott, 2015; Topping, Holmes, & Brenner, 2000) and social skills programs for students with autism and genetic disorders are recommended (Laugeson et al., 2015; Muldoon et al., 2015). However, these practices are not connected to specific brain processes. Rehabilitation psychologists have studied pro-social and anti-social behaviors in children with brain trauma and report that interventions focused on specific skills retraining in "real-world" situations are efficacious. Individuals with brain damage recover trained skills more quickly and consistently than they recover spontaneous, appropriate, social, and adaptive behavior (Park & Ingles, 2001). Although early adolescent anti-social actions have been linked to poor social skill development, studies showing anomalies in brain development have not been found. However, the field of social neuroscience is growing and researchers are making efforts to link diagnostic markers to intervention and treatment efforts.

Self-Esteem and Self-Efficacy

There is an extensive body of research on self-concept development, especially in relation to self-esteem (i.e., a positive global evaluative sense of self). The concept of self-efficacy (i.e., having a sense of agency regarding one's ability to achieve specific goals), discussed by Bandura (1997), has received increasing attention. Research on the "self" has been theoretically based, relying primarily on observational and self-report data, but it has not been linked to brain research. Studies have noted that areas in the brain are activated differentially when success or failure follows an effort or when there are perceptions of approval or disapproval from others. Also, children may feel more effective and may receive more positive feedback from others as neural pathways become strengthened or expanded in developmentally appropriate ways. Presently, however, the debate about whether first getting positive feedback that then results in efficacy feelings or having successful experiences that then affect one's global sense of self cannot be answered by brain research.

Standards-Based Education/Curriculum Alignment

Because evidence suggests that schooling affects brain growth and neurological development, emphasis on standards-based education and curriculum alignment with state proficiency tests may have an impact on the brain, especially when pruning begins in earnest. Ways of thinking that assist children in performing well on such tests may be strengthened as pruning occurs and those skills that are practiced in schools may remain across the lifespan. No longitudinal studies of brain changes resulting from certain school practices, such as curriculum alignment with tests, have been undertaken. Some educators are concerned that an excessive focus on standards-based information and frequent testing may negatively affect brain processes, but at present there is no evidence. It is likely that memory pathways are affected by the educational focus of the curriculum, and these effects may be both positive and negative. The other potential effect of such practices, however, may be on social and emotional development. Reports of children staying home on test days occurs as some parents see the testing as harmful for their children's development.

Whole Language/Phonics Training

Although debates over extremes of these two practices still rage occasionally, most educators acknowledge that both are useful for helping children learn to read and that "educational approaches that fail to include all aspects are misguided" (Byrnes & Vu, 2015, p. 9). Brain research on individuals with learning disabilities provides clues that might guide educational practice (Shaywitz & Shaywitz, 2013). Research on the general structures and functions of the brain suggests that children must have both the ability to put together specifics of sound/symbol correspondence (bottom-up approach) and meaning-making strategies promoted by whole language or balanced literacy (top-down approach), although the processes involved in these approaches may be sited in different areas of the brain. Because the brain operates as an integrated whole, children must incorporate all these skills to become readers. Educators' roles involve understanding why children have difficulty making sense of phonics, whole language, vocabulary, fluency, or comprehension instruction, and providing targeted scaffolding to encourage development of the skills that are missing.

Mindfulness

Stemming from Dewey's (1938) focus on the embodied experiences of learning, mindfulness is an area of practice gaining traction in schools. As a component of social-emotional learning, mindfulness has been reported to reduce negative behaviors, increase social-emotional competencies, improve attitudes and emotional regulation, and increase academic success (Berto & Barbiero, 2014). While best practices have yet to be established, implementation of various mindfulness practices are reported to have had positive effects on the brain and behavior of some children. Some mindfulness practices undertaken by children and adolescents have promoted long-lasting attentional control, reduced social anxiety and depression, and increased emotional regulation (Sanger & Dorjee, 2015). Mindfulness interventions require educators and clinicians to be active practitioners. Such contemplative practices are now considered important for maintaining a healthy brain, although conclusive brain research on specifics of this practice is not available.

Environmental Education

Recently there has been renewed focus on environmental education and research is being conducted on the effects on children's health and attitude toward the environment. Such experiences may help develop children's capacity to think critically, creatively, and ethically, make informed decisions about sustaining and enhancing the natural environment, and act as change agents for the future. Most research does not discuss how nature affects brain development, however, although the human brain evolved in the natural world. Some studies report that proximity to trees enhances children's health, well-being, and school achievement, and that environmental education has positive effects on a child's understanding of STEM concepts (Erhabor & Don, 2016). Also, school gardens are popular and research is focused on how they may affect children's healthy eating and natural-world interactions (Crone & Dahl, 2012). While school gardens, outdoor learning, and forest schools are promising developments, starting and sustaining these efforts require substantial commitments of time, resources, and community involvement. Both practitioners and researchers can encourage natural-world experiences and study effects that such experiences have on brain development.

Implications of Brain Research for Advocacy of Excellence in Education and Clinical Practice

While brain research does not speak clearly to specific professional practices, it does speak to some advocacy issues of concern for educators, clinicians, other professionals, parents, and the general society, including the following.

Excellence of Prenatal Care

The importance of excellent prenatal care has been outlined in relation to brain growth and neurological development. The lack of such care is a global problem that can be attacked only by a concerted effort that draws all interested parties into the mix, including parents, parents-to-be, educators, medical personnel, government officials, and other concerned citizens. This is one area in which brain research is clear, although public policy indicates that early and effective prenatal care is still seen as an option rather than a necessity. Educators and other professionals should: (1) collaborate with health care professionals to reduce infant mortality and improve prenatal care; (2) work with parents and children in early education programs to foster knowledge dissemination and change; and (3) communicate with legislators and support worldwide organizations that provide information about the importance of prenatal care and provide funding to assist women to obtain it.

Quality Early Child Care and Education

Brain research findings lend support to calls for quality early child care and education programs. Other types of research also show that consistency of educarers and educators aids early attachment development and high-quality programs facilitate cognitive and social development, as well as greater effectiveness throughout life. While the exact nature of the links between brain growth and neurological development and high-quality care and education have not been directly studied, advocates for such programs can draw upon the brain research literature to strengthen their recommendations (Shonkoff & Philllips, 2000).

Safe Environments

Safe environments include conditions of both physical and social-emotional safety. Most researchers on brain development agree that social-emotional safety during the first years of a child's life, as well as throughout life, is important for healthy brain growth. Efforts to increase safe and health-promoting environments are needed worldwide. While some attention has been paid recently to preventing child abuse and neglect, there are still many children living in such conditions and many who are hypervigilant, fearful, and/or unable to concentrate on learning. Child abuse or neglect contributes to learning problems, poor brain growth, and negative neurological development. Thus, brain research evidence must lead the way in promoting safe environments for all children and adolescents throughout the world, and professionals can work with groups concerned about this issue to create such safe and enriched environments.

Knowledgeable Educators, Clinicians, and Other Professionals

Research shows that personnel who have knowledge of children's developmental needs and of methods for facilitating their development are better able to enhance developmental growth. No brain research has specifically evaluated brain growth and neurological development in relation to the educational level of personnel who work with children, but psychological and educational research has documented that well-informed individuals have more complex cognitive processes (Fischer, 2008). Research to explore the aspects of professional practice that best support children's neurological development is needed as well as parent education on supporting brain development.

Excellent Funding for Education at All Levels

If all individuals in a society are to be effective contributors to that society, they must have life conditions that foster optimal brain development. Therefore, to foster that societal goal, there must be a commitment to funding all education venues at excellent levels. It should not be the case that children who live in one area of the country should have educational venues that are well equipped with highly trained and well-paid educators, and those in other areas have poorer educational opportunities.

Conclusions

Although research has provided much information about the brain and processes involved in its growth and neurological development, this information is not yet well known by all professionals. Many current practices can be hypothesized as likely to affect brain structures and functions, but few have been validated by brain research. It is important that professionals involved in the care, education, and evaluation of children, youth, and adults understand brain research and evaluate claims for "brain-based" strategies. In some areas (e.g., prenatal and infancy) where research findings demonstrate potentially negative effects on the brain from poor environmental conditions, professionals should be advocates for improvement of such conditions. The authors agree with Thompson and Nelson (2001) that public information about the importance of prenatal care, early nutrition, immunizations, and elimination of environmental toxins must be made widely available because this information "may accomplish as much to promote early brain development as public information campaigns focusing on the significance of talking and singing to young infants" (p. 12).

Lichtman (2001) suggests that "educators are in essence brain engineers, applied scientists who could, in principle, use the available information as a means of informing their educational practice and policies" (p. 41). He calls on educators and other practitioners to communicate with neuroscientists because "contrary to the impression created by some media accounts, researchers are at the vanguard—not the end—of exciting new discoveries about brain development" (Thompson & Nelson, 2001, p. 12).

Study Guide/Questions for Discussion

- Interview two professionals in disciplines that should base practice on brain development knowledge and contrast the way they use (or do not use) this knowledge in their work.

- Create a campaign for the public that promotes some aspect of practice based on brain research. Describe the target population in need of this information.

Bibliography

Bailey, D. B., Bruer, J. T., Symons, F. J., & Lichtman, J. W. (Eds.). (2001). *Critical thinking about critical periods*. Baltimore, MD: Paul H. Brookes.

Bandura, A. (1997). *Self-efficacy: The exercise of control*. New York: Freeman.

Bergen, D., Davis, D., & Abbitt, J. (2016). *Technology play and brain development: Infancy to adolescence and future implications*. New York: Taylor & Francis.

Berto, R., & Barbiero, G. (2014). Mindful silence produces long lasting attentional performance in children. *Visions for Sustainability, 2*, 49–60.

Blakemore, S. J., & Robbins, T. W. (2012). Decision-making in the adolescent brain. *Nature Neuroscience, 15*(9), 1184–1191.

Bruner, J. S. (1964). The course of cognitive growth. *American Psychologist, 19*(1), 1–15. doi:10.1037/h0044160.

Byrnes, J. P., & Vu, L. T. (2015). Educational neuroscience: Definitional, methodological, and interpretive issues. *Wiley Interdisciplinary Reviews: Cognitive Science, 6*(3), 221–234.

Cairns, K. (2017). Connecting to food: Cultivating children in the school garden. *Children's Geographies, 15*(3), 304–318.

Courage, M. L., Bakhtiar, A., Fitzpatrick, C., Kenny, S., & Brandeau, K. (2015). Growing up multitasking: The costs and benefits for cognitive development. *Developmental Review*, 35, 5-41

Crone, E. A., & Dahl, R. E. (2012). Understanding adolescence as a period of social—affective engagement and goal flexibility. *Nature Reviews Neuroscience, 13*(9), 636–650.

Dehn, M. J. (2011). *Working memory and academic learning: Assessment and intervention*. New York; John Wiley & Sons.

Dewey, J. (1938). *Experience and education*. The Kappa Delta Phi Lecture Series–Collier Books.

Erhabor, N. I., & Don, J. U. (2016). Impact of environmental education on the knowledge and attitude of students towards the environment. *International Journal of Environmental and Science Education, 11*(12), 5367–5375.

Fischer, K. W. (2008). Dynamic cycles of cognitive and brain development: Measuring growth in mind, brain, and education. In A. M. Battro, K. W. Gischer, & P. Lena (Eds.), *The educated brain: Essays in neuroeducation* (pp. 127–150). Cambridge: Cambridge University Press.

Fuhrmann, D., Knoll, L. J., & Blakemore, S. J. (2015). Adolescence as a sensitive period of brain development. *Trends in Cognitive Sciences, 19*(10), 558–566.

Gardner, H. (2011). *Frames of mind: The theory of multiple intelligences*. New York: Basic Books.

Gardner, J., & Hott, B. L. (2015). Praise: An effective school-wide positive behavioral support tool. *The Journal of the Effective Schools Project, 22*, 41–45.

Gopnik, A., Meltzoff, A. N., & Kuhl, P. K. (1999). *The scientist in the crib: What early learning tells us about the mind*. New York: Harper-Collins.

Grey, I. M., Bruton, C., Honan, R., McGuinness, R., & Daly, M. (2007). Co-operative learning for children with an Autistic Spectrum Disorder (ASD) in mainstream and special class settings: An exploratory study. *Educational Psychology in Practice, 23*(4), 317–327.

Hallam, S. (2010). The power of music: Its impact on the intellectural, social and personal development of children and young people. *International Journal of Music Education, 28*(3), 269–289. doi:10.1177/025576140370658. http://ijm.sagepub.com.

Holmes, J., & Gathercole, S. E. (2014). Taking working memory training from the laboratory into the schools. *Educational Psychology, 34*(4), 440–450.

James, K. H., & Engelhardt, L. (2012). The effects of handwriting experience on functional brain development in pre-literate children. *Trends in Neuroscience and Education, 1*(1), 32-42.

Johnson, D. W., & Johnson, R. T. (1994). *Learning together and alone* (4th ed.). Boston, MA: Allyn and Bacon.

Kharitonova, M., Winter, W., & Sheridan, M. A. (2015). As working memory grows: A developmental account of neural bases of working memory capacity in 5-to 8-year old children and adults. *Journal of Cognitive Neuroscience, 27*(9), 1775–1788.

Kersey, A. J., & James, K. H. (2013). Brain activation patterns resulting from learning letter forms through active self-production and passive observation in young children. *Frontiers in Psychology, 4*(567). http://dx.doi.org/10.3389/fpsyg.2013.00567.

Knudsen, E. I. (2004). Sensitive periods in the development of the brain and behavior. *Journal of Cognitive Neuroscience, 16*(8), 1412–1425.

Kyndt, E., Raes, E., Lismont, B., Timmers, F., Cascallar, E., & Dochy, F. (2013). A meta-analysis of the effects of face-to-face cooperative learning: Do recent studies falsify or verify earlier findings? *Educational Research Review, 10*, 133–149.

Laugeson, E. A., Gantman, A., Kapp, S. K., Orenski, K., & Ellingsen, R. (2015). A randomized controlled trial to improve social skills in young adults with autism spectrum disorder: The UCLA PEERS® program. *Journal of Autism and Developmental Disorders, 45*(12), 3978–3989.

Lee, L. (2015). Young children, play, and technology: Meaningful ways of using technology and digital media. In D. P. Fromberg & D. Bergen (Eds.), *Play from birth to twelve* (3rd ed., pp. 217–224). New York: Routledge.

Lichtman, J. W. (2001). Developmental neurobiology overview: Synapses, circuits, and plasticity. In D. B. Bailey, J. T. Bruer, F. J. Symons, & J. W. Lichtman (Eds.), *Critical thinking about critical periods* (pp. 27–42). Baltimore, MD: Paul H. Brookes.

Mercer, N. (2013). The social brain, language, and goal-directed collective thinking: A social conception of cognition and its implications for understanding how we think, teach, and learn. *Educational Psychologist, 48*(3), 148–168.

Miller, G., Church, R., & Trexler, M. (2000). Teaching diverse learners using robotics. In A. Druin & J. Hendler (Eds.), *Robots for kids: Exploring new technologies for learning* (pp. 166–191). San Francisco, CA: Morgan Kaufmann.

Moreno, S., Bialystok, E., Barac, R., Schellenberg, E. G., Cepeda, N. J., & Chau, T. (2011). Short-term music training enhances verbal intelligence and executive function. *Psychological Science, 22*(11), 1425–1433. doi:10.1177/0956797611416999.

Muldoon, M., Ousley, O. Y., Kobrynski, L. J., Patel, S., Oster, M. E., Fernandez-Carriba, S., . . . Pearce, B. D. (2015). The effect of hypocalcemia in early childhood on autism-related social and communication skills in patients with 22q11 deletion syndrome. *European Archives of Psychiatry and Clinical Neuroscience, 265*(6), 519–524.

Omaha World Herald (Associated Press Report). (1999, May 6). Bach-a-bye baby: Academy gives classical music CDs to babies (p. 16-A).

Osterhout, L., Poliakov, A., Inoue, K., McLaughlin, J., Valentine, G., Pitkanen, I., . . . & Hirschensohn, J. (2008). Second-language learning and changes in the brain. *Journal of Neurolinguistics, 21*(6), 509-521

Panksepp, J. (1998). Attention deficit hyperactivity disorders, psychostimulants, and intolerance of childhood playfulness: A tragedy in the making? *Current Directions in Psychological Science*, 7(3), 91–98.

Park, N. W., & Ingles, J. L. (2001). Effectiveness of attention rehabilitation after an acquired brain injury: A meta-analysis. *Neuropsychology, 15*(2), 199–210.

Peijnenborgh, J. C., Hurks, P. M., Aldenkamp, A. P., Vles, J. S., & Hendriksen, J. G. (2016). Efficacy of working memory training in children and adolescents with learning disabilities: A review study and meta-analysis. *Neuropsychological Rehabilitation, 26*(5-6), 645–672.

Sanger, K. L., & Dorjee, D. (2015). Mindfulness training for adolescents: A neurodevelopmental perspective on investigating modifications in attention and emotion regulation using event-related brain potentials. *Cognitive, Affective, & Behavioral Neuroscience, 15*(3), 696–711.

Shaywitz, S. E., & Shaywitz, B. A. (2013). Making a hidden disability visible: What has been learned from the neurobiological studies of dyslexia. In H. L. Swanson, K. R. Harris, & S. Graham (Eds.), *Handbook of learning disabilities* (pp. 643–657). New York: Guilford.

Shonkoff, J. P., & Philllips, D. A. (Eds.). (2000). *From neurons to neighborhoods: The science of early childhood education.* Washington, DC: Institute of Medicine, National Academic Press.

Slavin, R. E. (1995). *Cooperative learning: Theory, research, and practice* (2nd ed.). Boston, MA: Allyn and Bacon.

Spear, L. P. (2013). Adolescent neurodevelopment. *Journal of Adolescent Health, 52*(2), S7–S13.

Summa-Chadwick, M. (2009). The power of music: The use of music protocols to enhance neurological function. *Exceptional Parent, 39*(7), 38–42.

Swanson, H. L. (2016). Working memory and strategy instruction in children with learning disabilities. In R. Schiff & R. M. Joshi (Eds.), *Interventions in learning disabilities* (pp. 227–241). New York: Springer International Publishing.

Sylwester, R. (1995). *A celebration of neurons: An educator's guide to the human brain.* Alexandria, VA: Association for Supervision and Curriculum Development.

Thompson, R. A., & Nelson, C. A. (2001). Developmental science and the media: Early brain development. *American Psychologist, 56*(1), 5–15.

Topping, K., Holmes, E. A., & Brenner, W. (2000). The effectiveness of school-based programs for the promotion of social competence. In R. Bar-On & J. Parker (Eds.), *The handbook of emotional intelligence: Theory, development, assessment, and application at home, school, and in the workplace* (pp. 411–432). San Francisco, CA: Jossey Bass.

Wan, C. Y., & Schlaug, G. (2010). Music making as a tool for promoting brain plasticity across the life span. *The Neuroscientist, 16*(5), 566–577.

Zakaria, E., Solfitri, T., Daud, Y., & Abidin, Z. Z. (2013). Effect of cooperative learning on Secondary school students' mathematics achievement. *Creative Education, 4*(2), 98.

Zeki, S. (2001). Artistic creativity and the brain. *Science, 293*(5527), 51–52.

Zentall, S. S., Kuester, D. A., & Craig, B. A. (2011). Social behavior in cooperative groups: Students at risk for ADHD and their peers. *The Journal of Educational Research, 104*(1), 28–41.

14

FUTURIST ISSUES AND PREDICTIONS FOR HUMAN BRAIN DEVELOPMENT

In his most recent book, E. O. Wilson (2016) takes note of the ongoing advances in artificial intelligences and "their multitudinous applications," which would have been considered "distantly futuristic a decade earlier" (p. 200). He goes on to say that the human brain "is not a product of engineering but of evolution" and so it is "jury-rigged," created through an evolutionary process, which enabled it to be "fitted by natural selection to the environment of the moment . . . (and, therefore) . . . the brain has evolved not so much as an organ of thought as an organ of survival" (p. 202).

There are many positive projections of cognitive and sensory capacity expansions in human brain capabilities in the future, most clearly described by futurists such as Ray Kurzweil (2005, 2014), who predicts that as various aspects of technology (e.g., "nanobots") augment the human brain, technology-augmented humans will become new creatures, ones who have much longer lives and even, perhaps, ones who may never die! Kurzweil predicts that in the next 20 years, nanobots inserted in human brains will be able to connect directly to the Cloud and thus humans will have much more brain power. Because these nanobots will have unlimited programming capabilities, they will give humans more sensory experiences and there will be "an explosion of knowledge." According to Scott (2014), these new technologies may be able to solve some of humankind's pervasive problems such as world hunger, and might reverse aging and even free humans from having to work (what he terms as an "archaic idea").

In a recent issue of *Popular Science* (Dec. 2016) entitled "The New Artificial Intelligence," experts made predictions about how various forms of technology may positively affect aspects of human life. For example, proliferation of "trained" robots and super-intelligent machines, major advances in medical practice focused on brain monitoring and functioning, scientific explorations of the universe and of the microbiotic world, new models of performance in art and other creative fields, and many changes in aspects of everyday life will be observed in this rapid and pervasive technological revolution. These potentially wide-ranging effects are being proposed and discussed, but they are not yet being fully explored. However, within the lifetimes of present-day humans, many of these predictions, as well as other non-predicted changes, will probably be realized.

For educators, clinicians, parents, and others who are concerned with human brain development, alternative "thinking" machines are both promising and concerning, especially because they have observed how some aspects of present-day technology-augmented experiences already negatively affect common educational, clinical, and child-rearing practice. As Wilson has suggested, human brains will adapt to these changes not only because they are "organs of thought" but also because they are "organs of survival." How these adaptations will change the survival capabilities of the human brain is presently only speculation. However, there certainly will be effects on brain development, and thus on health, education, social interactions, government, science, and art, as well as on future technologies. As these technologies become more and more pervasive, future developmental researchers must observe and determine how the replacement or diminishment of human-to-human direct interaction with greater virtual or other technology-augmented interaction may create differences in the brains of humans, and thus change both the brain's developmental trajectory and its ultimate state.

Potential Impact of New Technologies on Human Brain Development

Since all experiences have the potential to affect human brain development, new technologies may also have effects at every age level.

Prenatal

The prenatal world already has been affected by various medical technologies that have enabled pregnancies to be assisted, sex characteristics to be determined, and diagnoses of fetal disease conditions and other teratogens (e.g., drug use) to be observed before birth. Recently, Sayres and Cho (2011) have noted that identification and analysis of cell-free fetal DNA and RNA is now possible, with the ability to detect single-gene disorders, chromosomal abnormalities, and fetal inheritance of other diseases and conditions. Such practices may result in improving fetal brain development. However, while such prenatal screening procedures will provide much important information, these authors note that there will be "significant ethical, legal, and social questions" (p. 31) that will be raised and need to be addressed by users of these technologically advanced diagnostic procedures. More questions will occur with the potential use of other types of fetal technology. For example, the use of fetal stem cells as a source for heart value tissue engineering (Schmidt et al., 2008); the determination of fetal brain abnormalities with ultrasound (Rizzo et al., 2011); and the conducting of fetal surgery (inside the mother) (Williams, 2006) all pose both practical and ethical dilemmas, with possible unexpected side effects of these technologies. A current example involves assisted reproductive technology, which has resulted in disproportionate levels of very-low-birth-weight infants in the United States, and such infants often have developmental problems (Schieve et al., 2002). According to Savage and colleagues (2011), such infants are "phenotypically and biochemically different from naturally conceived children" (p. 1) and they may be more prone to certain diseases. An important philosophical issue also has been raised: the technologies focused on the fetus are implicitly raising assumptions that the fetus is a being separate from the mother and the woman is merely the carrying body for the fetus (Williams, 2006). This perspective implies that the mother is "principally a generative space" (Williams, 2006, p. 1700), which was the view of Aristotle! Whether such ideas will ultimately result in technologically designed "generative spaces" for fetal growth rather than having women provide that space is presently unknown. Perhaps the future will hold some version of Huxley's "Brave New World" (1931) in which fetal growth was controlled scientifically.

Infancy

Presently there are indications that young children are being exposed to virtual devices and technologically-augmented toys that call for responsive interactions that are different from those infants and toddlers experienced in the past. A few researchers are already noting differences in both infant/parent and toddler play with such devices (Bergen et al., 2010; Smith, 2002). The possible effects of such changes in play behaviors and parent/child interactions on infant brain development is not presently known. However, there is theoretical evidence that the effects may be profound. The study of infant cognition has been extensive since the publication of Piaget's (1945) observations of his own young children and his descriptions of the cognitive schema being developed in the predominantly sensorimotor-focused first two years of life. He asserted that these interactions in the infancy period provided the foundation for all later cognition, and he described many ways that infants were "thinking in action." Building on Piagetian theory, Bruner (1964) termed early sensorimotor-based thought as "enactive cognition" and stated that this type of cognition was essential for the later development of "iconic" (image-related) and "symbolic" (arbitrary symbols) thought levels. Recently, Liu and colleagues (2008), who studied brain wave patterns in sensorimotor areas of the brains of infants, stated that developmental theorists and researchers have confirmed that "quality sensory input and appropriate motor responses are crucial during the period when infants are forming schema about their world" and they agree with earlier theorists that such early schema are "critical to the development of thought and language" (p. 43).

Researchers who focus on the study of "mirror neurons" also have confirmed that when infant/adult socially playful interactions occur, these neurons are especially active and may be predictive of later social attachments (Saby, Meltzoff, & Marshall, 2013). Although there is not yet evidence of what the brain development effects of infants' extensive interactions with technology-augmented toys or virtual realities will be, it is plausible that if such "iconic" interactions replace "enactive" cognition, then the brains of infants and the quality of children's later cognitive development will be influenced. It is too early to predict that these changes will be harmful as perhaps they will better prepare infants for this technology-augmented future world. There is no question that their brain development will be influenced, however, because, as the Hindu saying reminds us, for the child, "Everything is food."

Early Childhood

As noted earlier, the early childhood age period is one in which an explosion of synaptic connections occurs in the brain. Observers of children of this age often note that they seem to learn something new every day. That rapid brain growth is demonstrated both in the children's cognitive elaboration of actions and in their demonstrations of greater language competence. Comparatively, this period of childhood has typically been a time in which rich, complex, and primarily child-generated play themes occur. Traditional play materials, such as blocks, replica objects (e.g., cars and trucks, dolls, animal figures), and large muscle/outdoor play objects (e.g., climbers, tricycles) suggest actions but allow a wide range of interactive behaviors. Technologically-augmented devices now are pervasive in the lives of young children, and most of these devices give clear messages about the expected behaviors children should use to activate and respond to them. There are varied opinions of both short-term and long-term effects of such play materials. Goldstein (2013) notes that since toys have always been the medium through which children learn about the values and practices of their culture, they now learn that cultural information within a technology-augmented environment. Levin (2013) states, however, that these cultural messages may not be appropriate for children because many are gender stereotypic, violent, or draw on other negative aspects of the culture. Kafai (2006) indicates that technology-augmented play can be a new type of "playground" for today's children but she recommends that these materials include programmable blocks, computational games, and virtual playgrounds that include constructive activities. One present example of such a virtual playground is "Minecraft."™ Jenkins et al. (2009) has stated that skills being learned through technology-augmented play are important ones that will be needed in future work settings. Research on the effects of early technology-augmented play is sparse but generally supports the perspective that such toys have greater control over the themes and actions observed in the child's play than do older types of toys (see Bergen, 2007; Marsh, 2010). That is, the toys "act" and the child "reacts." Although longitudinal effects of technology-augmented play materials are not yet known, it is reasonable to conclude that children may gain more sophisticated and future-oriented, less developmentally appropriate, or just different behaviors and messages from their play with technology-augmented devices than they gained from more traditional toys.

Another potential effect of the pervasive technology-augmented toy environment is that it may diminish the amount of time that adults and older children spend in socially rich activities with young children. Because every age level of persons in a family may focus on their own technology-augmented devices, they may give less attention to activities that typically have involved both child and adult interaction, such as book reading, block building, and board games, which in past generations contributed to the socialization and learning of young children. Thus, social relationship knowledge may not be the same as that learned in the past. When face-to-face playful interactions with other people are replaced by interactions on technologically-augmented devices, different social behaviors may be the ones practiced. Kahn and colleagues (2004), after a study of preschool children's play with a robotic toy, reported that the play had resulted in "impoverished" social relationships. Although this concern has been expressed by some developmental theorists, there are few studies that have discussed the potential long-term consequences on brain development of fewer adult/child play interactions and more technology/child play interactions during this age period. It may be that these technology-influenced childhood experiences may prepare young children's brains better for the future world they will encounter, while at the same time reducing many of the "survival brain" skills that were useful in the past.

Elementary, Middle Childhood, and Adolescent Age Levels

Because brain maturation continues throughout elementary, middle childhood, and adolescent years, and more individualization of brain structures occurs as children's experiences become more focused, based on their interests and opportunities, interactions with technology-augmented devices also will influence brain development during this age period. The brain's frontal lobe is at its highest synaptic density at about age 7, and for the next 10–15 years pruning of less often used connections and strengthening of highly used connections occurs extensively. Thus, it is possible that technological advances related to learning, communication, and socialization are likely to influence the final structures of these children's brains. Thompson and Nelson (2001) have stated that brain areas such as the insula, amygdala, and hippocampus, which are involved in reasoning, problem-solving, and self-regulation, take a long time to mature and their maturation is not completed until late adolescence; thus, interactions with technology-augmented devices during childhood and adolescence may particularly affect the maturation of those brain areas. For example, the ready availability of GPS systems already may be affecting development of geographic spatial knowledge features and the instant availability of information on the internet may be influencing memory storage abilities. Of course, past technological inventions also influenced brain development. The invention of writing and reading reduced the need for extensive factual memory capacity (Foer, 2011). Because technology-augmented devices are prevalent in both educational settings and out-of-school activities, it seems reasonable to assume that the types and amounts of technologically-augmented experiences that young individuals have will influence specific brain maturation patterns, especially those related to cognitive and social-emotional skills that mature over long time periods.

Designers of formal learning experiences now use many technology-augmented methods, and personnel from schools and colleges integrate online learning experiences into the curriculum. Although such methods may be effective, especially for learning routine and factual knowledge, research on long-term effectiveness is sparse. According to Coates and colleagues (2005), such technology-augmented innovations are likely to have long-term effects on teaching processes, student engagement, the nature of academic work, and ultimately the control of knowledge. Many technologically-based curriculum materials use strategies such as game-based learning, game design, and gamification, and these may be effective in engaging students as well as in enhancing higher-order learning. However, most designers of technology-augmented learning experiences have little knowledge of the brain development trajectory of children and adolescents, and thus, even if these experiences are motivating and use creative methods for presenting knowledge, because collaboration with scholars who understand developmental learning processes is limited and there is little research on possible effects of technology-augmented learning on brain development, long-term effects of such learning methods on brain development could be problematic.

There are also concerns expressed about the non-school pervasiveness of virtual media in the lives of children and adolescents. Juvonen and Gross (2008) have studied bullying and social exclusion that occurs on various social media used by children in this age range. They suggest that children have more difficulty in evaluating potential social effects of virtual media comments and responses than in understanding face-to-face social interactions. Bauerlein (2008) has noted that some adolescents have contracted their range of face-to-face and embodied cognition experiences because they spend most of their time in their own virtual world of gaming and social media, and thus they risk becoming isolated from the larger culture. There is an addictive quality to virtual experiences so they have the potential to displace all other activities, especially those that involve the broader physical world. Human brain development will certainly be affected if the balance of enactive and virtual experiences changes, since the brain's mature structure is derived from the diversity and depth of each human's total life experiences. Conversely, if children and adolescents are participants in opportunities to design technology-augmented experiences, such as computer programs and virtual learning devices, these creative technology activities might extend and enrich human brain maturation in positive ways (Resnick, 2006). If interactive experiences designing and using technology are incorporated in education, children and adolescents may be more prepared to have creative and productive lives in a technology-augmented world

Young and Middle Adult Age Level

Many issues that may affect brain development of children and adolescents also are relevant for adult brain development, especially for young adult brain development, since there are important developmental changes occurring in the brains of individuals under 30. Many young adults now spend much time in virtual interactions, with smart phones, virtual games, social media, and other technologically-augmented activities. Even sports training now may include practice with eye-tracking video games designed to enhance performance (Schonbrun, 2017). Young adult employment responsibilities also involve the use of devices related to technological innovations. Potential addiction of young adults to the use of such devices may result in both positive and negative long-term brain development for themselves. For example, they may work more effectively in technology-oriented occupations and create many innovative devices using this knowledge themselves. If so, the synaptic areas of their brains that are stimulated by these different activities will be strengthened and they may be more prepared to use and benefit from the technology-augmented world. However, if they also spend less time in "real-world" activities—that is, those that do not involve virtual worlds—they may lose some skills that were valued in earlier times, as has been the case whenever a pervasive technological change has occurred. Many skills adults had in the past (e.g., driving horse-drawn buggies, knitting hats, sewing shirts and dresses, digging ditches, and even doing routine factory jobs) are now rarely used because other technologies have made those skills less needed.

Since young adults also are the primary group involved in raising young children, if their use of such technology-augmented devices changes their interactive behaviors with their children, the behavioral changes also may affect the brain development of children. For example, if they primarily give their children technology-augmented playthings and activities, and if their own engagement and time is consumed with experiences involving these technologies, it may result in different parent/child interaction patterns. Both parents and children may spend more time using these devices, reducing engagement in adult/child interactive talk, social games, large motor play, and outdoor activities. Thus, there may be brain development consequences for both parents and children. Presently there are no longitudinal research studies and few short-term research studies that address these questions. It will be important for developmental researchers to study long-term effects of the impact of advanced technologies on the brain development not only of children, but also of adults of all ages. As further advances in brain science and a plethora of inventions of new technological instruments for both learning and play become available, they will certainly affect how human brains adapt to survive and prosper in the future technology-augmented world.

Older Adult Age Level

Recent research has shown that there is great variation in the brain health of older adults. Those who encounter a major illness, especially one that has consequences for brain developmental health, often lose significant executive control processes, such as memory, analytical ability, and even socioemotional control. However, other older adults maintain their clarity of thinking and other cognitive and socioemotional skills for many years. These differences have been of interest especially to developers of technological aids specifically designed to help older adults maintain and even increase their brain health. Recently, many technology-augmented devices have been promoted as ones that will improve the cognition of older adults, and there are questions about the effectiveness of such experiences. Kueider and colleagues (2012) reviewed 38 studies of computer-based cognitive interventions, including classic cognitive training tasks (21), neuropsychological software interventions (9), and video game interventions (8) to gain information on the effectiveness of such procedures. They concluded, "all three approaches to computerized training . . . appear to hold promise for improving cognitive abilities in cognitively normal, community dwelling older adults who have a high risk of cognitive decline as they age" (p. 10). The researchers state that the older adults who benefitted were not "technologically savvy" but they quickly learned and seemed to enjoy these computer-generated experiences. Another recent study of cognitive control processes involved in multitasking (Anguera et al., 2013) showed that, although multitasking performance in a 3-D video game typically shows a linear age-related decline (from age 2 to age 79), an adaptive version of the game, used with adults ages 60 to 85, increased their ability to multitask and sustain attention and that the improvement was still evident six months later. They concluded that the training showed that there is "robust plasticity of the prefrontal cognitive control system in the aging brain" (p. 1) and suggest that video games can both assess and improve cognitive enhancement at later age levels. The studies did not include individuals with cognitive impairments, but it is likely that such training might delay cognitive decline in older adults who begin to have cognitive impairments.

A recent article in the New York Times (Gustke, 2017) stated that another technology-augmented area that will be likely to affect older adult brain development is that of "consumer robotics." Within the next five years, older adults may have robots do most of the work of caregivers (e.g., laundry, cleaning, personal care) and their cost will be about 20% of the present cost of a caregiver. Some testing of robots in retirement communities shows that older adults interact well with them and are gaining life enhancements through being able to "take trips" by viewing other places through virtual reality devices and to stay in touch with family members with video calls. Thus, social aspects of brain health may be enhanced with such devices. Presently there is great interest in technology-augmented experiences for older adults since they are becoming a larger share of the world population. One interesting issue is whether the aging population in the future will have less cognitive decline because they were avid technology-users in their youth and earlier adult lives, or whether their range of cognitive and social skills will be narrower because of their earlier intense focus on technology-augmented devices and their lifelong engagement with such devices.

Potential Impact of Human Brain Developmental Change on General Life Experiences

One interesting aspect of the increase in technological sophistication is in advances being made in problematic areas of human development due to these new devices. While many technological advances point to positive results such as those predicted by Kursweil, they also may raise issues related to Wilson's concerns. Thus, health and longevity, social-emotional interactions, political and government practices, and science and art creations may be affected both positively and negatively by new technological advances. Whether they ultimately will increase or decrease the human brain's survival skills is presently an open question.

Health and Longevity

Already there are positive health-related examples of the brain-technology interface, such as the use of nanoparticle technology for more effective drug delivery to patients (Lockman et al., 2002), improvements in neurological rehabilitation (Dobkin, 2006), and successes in brain stimulation therapy (Fregni & Pascual-Leon, 2007). There also are predictions of how brain-computer interface technology methods may enhance aspects of brain/body functioning (e.g., Millan et al., 2010). For example, Sas and Chopra (2015) discuss a type of wearable neurofeedback-based system focused on enhancing mindfulness that seems to have benefits, particularly for novice meditators. Technological innovations may solve developmental problems related to disabilities. For example, Allievi and colleagues (2014) reported that neuroimaging of the sensorimotor functioning of infant brains may enable early diagnosis and effective treatment of diseases such as cerebral palsy.

Science and Art

Scientific research and product development has been greatly affected by the possibilities of technologically-enhanced methods. Such technologies have influenced biological, physical, chemical, and other fields of science in the past, as well as specific scientific disciplines, such as microelectronics, material science, polymer science, aerospace, and forensic science. According to Klein and colleagues (2012), however, although specific scientific areas have informed societal knowledge systems, it is now crucial for both academics and practitioners to engage in "transdisciplinary" science to solve problems in the future. These scientists suggest that interdisciplinary scientific work will be most needed in the future. In a working paper on the future of the science-technology-innovation complex, Freeman and Soete (2007) note that the continuously and rapidly evolving status of this complex is not similar to the past. They state that "frontiers and characteristics that were important last century may no longer be so relevant today and indeed may even be positively misleading" (p. 3). Where these new transdisciplinary approaches will lead is presently unknown, and thus, their effects on brain development are also unknown.

The visual and performing art worlds always have embraced the latest technology. For example, composers incorporated new string, woodwind, and other instruments into their compositions and painters used varied types of paint and drawing techniques that became available with technological improvements. Digital technology has now greatly affected the arts (Candy & Edmonds, 2012; Wands, 2007). Wands discusses the radical transformations in more traditional art forms, such as drawing, painting, and sculpture, and states that new media are pushing past boundaries of what art can be due to the inclusion of these technologically-augmented materials. Some artists are also using art to make statements about issues of social and political natures. Similarly, musical expression has been transformed by recent technological devices such as analog synthesizers, computer creation and editing, and electronic performance. Holmes (2012) states, "what was once an exclusively experimental kind of musical expression formed a foundation on which nearly every familiar genre of music has since constructed a room of its own" (p. XIV). Artistic performance seems more accessible to the general population, as artistic contests and open-mike performances demonstrate. Although some art lovers are concerned that more traditional performances may disappear, at least at present, they are still available for those who support them, although the continuing existence of earlier art and music forms may wane as technology-augmented art becomes dominant.

Social Interactions, Politics, and Government

Potential effects of technological change on brains and resulting changes in human social interactions may have effects on many aspects of social interactions, as well as on political and governmental institutions. On an individual level, researchers studying violent video game usage already have reported that high levels of use of video-game play increases aggression-related thoughts and feelings and decreases pro-social behaviors among such individuals (Anderson & Bushman, 2001). There is also the likelihood that, as older adults' positive interactions with robots suggest, robotic helpers who become human companions may replace face-to-face human social interactions. Presently, there is no research on these potential long-term effects.

Because technology-augmented communication now connects the entire world, there are both positive and negative worldwide effects reported. Positively, such communication can draw people from many parts of the world together and enhance social and cognitive understanding. However, more problematic possibilities are also evident. Technology-augmented communication devices (e.g., *Facebook*, *Twitter*) may affect citizens' understanding of social and political issues because these communication methods have empowered various groups who can directly reach potential followers, raise funds for political causes, increase fervor of beliefs about issues, and encourage their believers to vote for certain candidates or support certain government policies. These accessible technological communication devices also are changing perceptions of what is legitimate news and what are "alternative facts" (a newly coined term). That is, communication about information and issues is no longer the purview of recognized journalistic news sources that follow ethical journalism guidelines. In early 2017, it was reported that the book *1984* (Orwell, 1949), in which "newspeak" (fake news) controls public opinion, has again become a "best seller" because it addresses issues of information control that are relevant in part because of the effects of popularized technology-augmented sources of information (Andrews, 2017).

Another area of concern is that easy access to communication devices with revolutionary themes has caused radicalization of many young people and adults, some of whom have then become terrorists, resulting in grave consequences for countries throughout the world (Lennings et al., 2010). There is now greater concern related to the likelihood of potential attacks on the critical infrastructure and defense systems of various countries by technologically sophisticated groups intent on harming those in other societies (Makhutov, 2009). These are just two examples of how the brain's social-emotional belief systems related to group membership can be affected by technologically-augmented communication. Group membership loyalty is one type of survival mechanism that has evolved in the human brain over time. Such group membership can be highly influenced by websites that stress varied world-views and thus, these communications can result in social and anti-social actions required by group membership maintenance. The long-range effects of the explosion of technologically-augmented communication on human social group memberships and belief systems are presently unknown.

Potential Impact of Future Technologies on Clinical and Educational Practices

It is often the case that when newer technologies are invented, there are dire predictions of problems and even active resistance to these changes. Presently, the loss of factory jobs to robotic workers is a major topic of conversation in the U.S.

However, this phenomenon is not a new one. A recent article in the *Smithsonian* magazine (Thompson, 2017) discusses how, in the early 1800s, workers in Britain rebelled against the technology of that time, automated cotton-weaving machines, which was causing them to lose their jobs. These "Luddites" staged attacks in which they broke the new machines and, when owners retaliated, more violence occurred. Thompson states that the fight was really about the fact that although the new technology provided greater productivity and resulted in financial gains, they "enriched only the machines' owners and weren't shared with the workers" (p. 23). The issue of who gains from advances in technology and who loses is one that is of present concern to many people.

How such future technological changes will affect clinical and educational practice is already of concern to practitioners. For example, online education is changing both the role and the potential financial health of teachers, and robotic caregivers and therapists are beginning to transform clinical practice. There will undoubtedly be new roles for human educators and clinicians, but presently this is an area of "terra incognita." Thus, the visions of futurists such as Kurzweil and biologists such as Wilson may both inform the technology-augmented future. It is vitally important that educators and clinicians have a solid knowledge of brain development and the effect of experiences on that development so that they can promote experiences that will enhance both optimum brain development and the future of humanity.

Study Guide/Questions for Discussion

- Read two articles that discuss potential effects on brain development of future technological changes on society. Critique the arguments presented and predict brain development changes that might occur at some age level if these changes occur.
- Plan a longitudinal research study on some aspect of brain development that might be affected by future societal changes.

Bibliography

Allievi, A. G., Arichi, T., Gordon, A. L., & Burdet, E. (2014). Technology-aided assessment of sensorimotor function in early infancy. *Frontiers in Neurology, 5*, 1–10. doi:10.3389/fneur.2014.00197.

Anderson, C. A., & Bushman, B. J. (2001). Effects of violent video games on aggressive behavior, aggressive cognition, aggressive affect, physiological arousal, and prosocial behavior: A meta-analytic review of the scientific literature. *Psychological Science, 12*(5), 353-359.

Andrews, T. M. (2017, January 25). Sale of Orwell's '1984' spike after Kellyanne Conway's 'alternative facts'. *The Washington Post*. Retrieved from www.washingtonpost.com/news/mornng.

Anguera, J. A., Boccanfuso, J., Rintoul, J. L., Al-Hashimi, O., Faraji, F., Janowich, J., Kong, E., Larraburo, Y., Rolle, C., Johnston, E., & Gazzaley, A. (2013). Video game training enhances cognitive control in older adults. *Nature, 501*(7465), 97-101

Bauerlein, M. (2008). *The dumbest generation: How the digital age stupefies young Americans and jeopardizes our future (or, don't trust anyone under 30).* New York: Penguin.

Bergen, D. (2007). Communicative actions and language narratives in preschoolers' play with "talking" and "non-talking" rescue heroes. In O. Jarrett & D. Sluss (Eds.), *Play investigations in the 21st century (Play and Culture Series,* Vol. 7, J. Johnson, Series ed., pp. 229–248). Lanham, MD: University Press of America.

Bergen, D., Hutchinson, K., Nolan, J., & Weber, D. (2010). Effects of infant-parent play with a technology-enhanced toy: Affordance related action and communicative interaction. *Journal of Research in Childhood Education, 24*(1), 1–17.

Bruner, J. S. (1964). The course of cognitive growth. *American Psychologist, 19*(1), 1–15.

Candy, L., & Edmonds, E. (2012). *Explorations in art and technology*. Berlin: Springer Science & Business Media.

Coates, H., James, R., & Baldwin, G. (2005). A critical examination of the effects of learning management systems on university teaching and learning. *Tertiary Education and Management, 11*, 19–36.

Dobkin, B. H. (2005). Rehabilitation after stroke. *New England Journal of Medicine, 352*(16), 1677-1684.

Foer, J. (2011). *Moonwalking with Einstein: The art and science of remembering everything.* New York: Penguin.

Freeman, C., & Soete, L. (2007). Science, technology and innovation indicators: The twenty-first century challenges. *Science, technology and innovation indicators in a changing world responding to policy needs: Responding to policy needs* (p. 271). OECD Blue Sky II Forum (Ottawa, Canada, 25–27 September 2006).

Fregni, F., & Pascual-Leone, A. (2007). Technology insight: noninvasive brain stimulation in neurology--perspectives on the therapeutic potential of rTMS and tDCS. Nature Reviews. *Neurology, 3*(7), 383.

Goldstein, J. H. (2013). Technology and play. *Scholarpedia, 8*(2), 30434. Scholarpedia. doi:10.4249/scholarpedia.30434.

Goodman, S. E., Kirk, J. C., & Kirk, M. H. (2007). Cyberspace as a medium for terrorists. *Technological Forecasting and Social Change*, 74(2), 193–210.

Gustke, C. (2017, Janurary 22). Retiring: Seniors welcome new, battery-powered friends. *The New York Times*, p. BU 5.

Hackett, E. J., Amsterdamska, O., Lynch, M., & Wajcman, J. (2008). *The handbook of science and technology studies*. Cambridge, MA: The MIT Press.

Holmes, T. (2012). *Electronic and experimental music: Technology, music, and culture*. New York: Routledge.

Huxley, A. (1931). *Brave new world*. New York: Harpers

Jenkins, H., Purushotma, R., Weigel, M., Clinton, K., & Robison, A. J. (2009). *Confronting the challenges of participatory culture: Media education for the 21st century*. Cambridge, MA: MIT Press.

Juvonen, J., & Gross, E. F. (2008). Extending the school grounds? Bullying experiences in cyberspace. *Journal of School Health*, 78(9), 496–505.

Kafai, Y. (2006). Play and technology: Revised realities and potential perspectives. In D. P. Fromberg & D. Bergen (Eds.), *Play from birth to twelve: Contexts, perspectives, and meanings* (2nd ed., pp. 207–214). New York: Routledge.

Kahn Jr., P. H., Friedman, B., Perez-Granados, D. R., & Freier, N. G. (2004, April). Robotic pets in the lives of preschool children. In *CHI'04 extended abstracts on human factors in computing systems*, ACM (pp. 1449–1452).

Klein, J. T., Grossenbacher-Mansuy, W., Häberli, R., Bill, A., Scholz, R. W., & Welti, M. (Eds.). (2012). *Transdisciplinarity: Joint problem solving among science, technology, and society: An effective way for managing complexity*. Switzerland: Birkhäuser.

Kueider, A. M., Parisi, J. M., Gross, A. L., & Rebok, G. W. (2012). Computerized cognitive training with older adults: A systematic review. *PloS One*, 7(7), e40588.

Kurzweil, R. (2005). *The singularity is near: When humans transcend biology*. New York: Penguin.

Kurzweil, R. (2014). The Singularity Is Near. In Sandler, R. (Ed.). *Ethics and Emerging Technologies*, pp. 393-406. London: Palgrave

Lennings, C. J., Amon, K. L., Brummert, H., & Lennings, N. J. (2010). Grooming for terror: The Internet and young people. *Psychiatry, Psychology and Law*, *17*(3), 424–437.

Levin, D. (2013). *Beyond remote-controlled childhood: Teaching young children in the media age*. Washington, DC: NAEYC.

Liu, W. C., Flax, J. F., Guise, K. G., Sukul, V., & Benasich, A. A. (2008). Functional connectivity of the sensorimotor area in naturally sleeping infants. *Brain Research*, *1223*, 42–49.

Lockman, P. R., Mumper, R. J., Khan, M. A., & Allen, D. D. (2002). Nanoparticle technology for drug delivery across the blood-brain barrier. *Drug Development and Industrial Pharmacy*, *28*(1), 1-13.

Makhutov, N. A., Petrov, V. P., & Reznikov, D. O. (2009, March). Characteristics of technological terrorism scenarios and impact factors. In *Countering Terrorism: Biological Agents, Transportation Networks, and Energy Systems* (*Summary of a US-Russian Workshop*, National Academy of Sciences, Washington, DC).

Marsh, J. (2010). Young children's play in online virtual worlds. *Journal of Early Childhood Research*, *8*(1), 23–39. doi:10.1177/1476718X09345406.

Millán J. d. R., Buttfield A., Vidaurre C., Krauledat M., Schögl A., Shenoy P., Blankertz B., Rao R. P. N., Cabeza R., Pfurtscheller G., Müller K.-R. (2007). Adaptation in brain–computer interfaces. In Dornhege G., Hinterberger T., McFarland D., Millán J. d. R., Müller K.-R. (Eds). *Toward Brain–Computer Interfacing*, pp. 303-325. Cambridge, MA: MIT Press.

Orwell, G. (1990). Nineteen Eighty-Four. 1949. *The Complete Novels*, 7. London: Penguin Books.

Piaget, J. (1945). *Play, dreams, and imitation in childhood*. London: Heinemann.

Plowman, L., & Luckin, R. (2004). Interactivity, interfaces, and smart toys. *Computer*, *37*(2), 98–100.

Resnick, M. (2006). Computer as paintbush: Tehnology, play, and the creative society. In D. G. Singer, R. M. Golinkoff, & K. Hirsh-Pasek (Eds.), *Play=learning: How play motivates and enhances children's cognitive and social-emotional growth*. New York: Oxford University Press.

Restivo, S. P. (2005). *Science, technology, and society: An encyclopedia*. Oxford: Oxford University Press on Demand.

Rizzo, G., Capponi, A., Pietrolucci, M. E., Capece, A., Aiello, E., Mammarella, S., & Arduini, D. (2011). An algorithm based on OmniView technology to reconstruct sagittal and coronal planes of the fetal brain from volume datasets acquired by three-dimensional ultrasound. *Ultrasound in Obstetrics & Gynecology*, *38*(2), 158–164.

Saby, J. N., Meltzoff, A. N., & Marshall, P. J. (2013). Infants' somatotopic neural responses to seeing human actions: I've got you under my skin. *PLoS One*, *8*(10), e77905.

Sas, C., & Chopra, R. (2015). MeditAid: A wearable adaptive neurofeedback-based system for training mindfulness state. *Personal and Ubiquitous Computing*, *19*(7), 1169–1182.

Savage, T., Peek, J., Hofman, P. L., & Cutfield, W. S. (2011). Childhood outcomes of assisted reproductive technology. *Human Reproduction*, *26*(9), 2392–2400. doi:10.1093/humrep/der212.

Sayres, L. C., & Cho, M. K. (2011). Cell-free fetal nucleic acid testing: A review of the technology and its applications. *Obstetrical & Gynecological Survey, 66*(7), 431–442.

Schieve, L. A., Meikle, S. F., Ferre, C., Peterson, H. B., Jeng, G., & Wilcox, L. S. (2002). Low and very low birth weight in infants conceived with use of assisted reproductive technology. *New England Journal of Medicine, 346*(10), 731–737.

Schmidt, D., Achermann, J., Odermatt, B., Genoni, M., Zund, G., & Hoerstrup, S. P. (2008). Cryopreserved amniotic fluid-derived cells: A lifelong autologous fetal stem cell source for heart valve tissue engineering. *The Journal of Heart Valve Disease, 17*(4), 446–55.

Schonbrun, Z. (2017, January 8). Honing 'gymnastics of the brain.' *The New York Times*, p SP 1, 4–5.

Scott, G. (2014). Visualizing the future. *The Futurist, 48*(4), 20–23.

Smith, C. R. (2002). Click on me! An example of how a toddler used technology in play. *Journal of Early Childhood Literacy, 2*(1), 5–20.

Thompson, O. (2017). Rage against the machines. *Smithsonian, 47*(9), 21–25.

Thompson, R. A., & Nelson, C. A. (2001). Developmental science and the media: Early brain development. *American Psychologist, 56*(1), 5–15.

Tyson, N. D. (2016). *Startalk radio show: A conversation with Ray Kurzweil.* Season 7: Episode 28.

Wands, B. (2007). *Art of the digital age.* New York: Thames & Hudson.

Williams, C. (2006). Dilemmas in fetal medicine: Premature application of technology or responding to women's choice? *Sociology of Health & Illness, 28*(1), 1–20.

Wilson, E. O. (2016). *Half-earth: Our planet's fight for life.* New York: W. W. Norton.

GLOSSARY OF BRAIN AND NERVOUS SYSTEM TERMS

Brain Components

Amygdala An almond-shaped mass of nuclei that form part of the gray matter in the front part of the temporal lobe; part of the limbic system; involved in processing and expressing emotions.

Basal ganglia A group of structures deep in the cerebral hemispheres involved in inhibition of motor movements.

Brain stem The section of the brain that includes the diencephalion (thalamus and hypothalamus), midbrain, and hindbrain.

Cerebellum A structure in the hindbrain specialized for motor coordination; also plays a role in learning and memory.

Cerebrum The rounded structure of the brain occupying most of the cranial cavity; divided into two hemispheres.

Corpus callosum The fiber system that connects the two hemispheres of the cerebrum.

Cortex The outer layer of the brain, containing four to six layers of cells.

Fissures Deep clefts produced by folds of the cortex.

Forebrain The portion of the brain that includes the cerebral hemispheres, basal ganglia, thalamus, amygdala, hippocampus, and septum.

Frontal lobe The portion of the cortex that is in front of the central sulcus.

Gyri Convolutions of the cortex in the cerebral hemispheres.

Hemisphere lateralization Specialization of functions in the two cerebral hemispheres.

Hindbrain The region of the brain that contains the cerebellum, medulla, pons, and fourth ventricle.

Hippocampus A structure in the anterior medial region of the temporal lobe involved in memory, learning, and emotions.

Hypothalamus A structure below the thalamus involved in behavior regulation (e.g., movement, feeding, sleeping, temperature, emotional expression, sexual activity, endocrine production).

Insula A portion of the cortex folded deep within the lateral sulcus involved in consciousness, emotion regulation, perception, motor control, self-awareness, other cognitive functions, and interpersonal experience.

Limbic system The neural systems on the inside wall of the cortex, surrounding the corpus callosum and brain stem, involved in learning, memory, and emotions.

Medulla The portion of the hindbrain near the spinal cord; regulates reflexes and blood pressure.

Midbrain The short segment between the forebrain and the hindbrain.

Occipital lobe The regions of the cortex at the back of the head; site of visual perception.

Parietal lobe The regions of the cortex lying beneath the parietal bone; site of motor and sensory perception.

Sulci Small clefts produced by the folding of the cortex.

Temporal lobes The regions of the cortex lying laterally on the sides of the head; site of language perception and speech.

Thalamus The structure that relays visual, auditory, and sensory information to and from the cortex.

Ventricles The cavities of the brain that contain cerebrospinal fluid.

Nervous System Components

Axon The part of the neuron that transmits action potentials from the cell body to other neurons, muscles, and glands.

CNS The central nervous system, including the brain and spinal cord.

Dendrites The treelike structures of the neuron that receive information from the axons of other neurons.

Efferent nerves Nerves that conduct impulses away from higher centers in the central nervous system toward muscles and glands.

Glia The brain cells that provide support for the neurons and central nervous system.

Myelination Formation of myelin coating on the axons; an index of brain maturation.

Neuron The basic unit of the nervous system, functioning to store and transmit information (includes cell body, dendrites, axon).

Neurotransmitters Chemicals released from synapses in response to action potentials; chemically transmit information from one neuron to another (e.g., cortisol, serotonin, dopamine).

Pruning The process by which excess synapses are eliminated.

Synapse The point where nerve cells make contact; junction between an axonal terminal and a dendrite of another cell.

Synaptogenesis The process by which synapses multiply.

INDEX

Page numbers in italic indicate a figure and page numbers in bold indicate a table.